Maryon Stewart studied preventive dentistry and nutrition at St George's Hospital in London and worked as a counsellor with nutritional specialists in England for four years. At the beginning of 1984 she set up the PMT Advisory Service, which has subsequently helped thousands of women worldwide. In 1987 she launched the Women's Nutritional Advisory Service, and the Natural Health Advisory Service (NHAS) in 2003, which provides broader help to both women and men of all ages.

Maryon Stewart is the author of 20 best-selling self-help books in the UK including *The Phyto Factor*, *Cruising through the Menopause*, *Beat Menopause Naturally* and *No More PMS*. She is the co-author of *No More IBS*, *Every Woman's Health Guide* and *The Natural Health Bible*.

Maryon Stewart has worked extensively on radio, including having her own weekly radio programme on health and nutrition, has co-written several medical papers and has written for many glossy magazines and for national daily newspapers. She has also appeared on many TV programmes on all five UK terrestrial channels, had a regular page in *House and Garden* and *Healthy Eating* and regular columns in the *Sunday Express Magazine* and the *Daily Mail*, has been both adviser and contributor to *Good Health Magazine*, on the Expert Panel for *Top Santé* magazine and *Health and Fitness Magazine* and currently writes for a variety of newspapers and magazines in the UK, USA and in Australia including the *Daily Express*, *OK* and *S*.

She appeared as the nutritional consultant for the Channel 4 programme *Model Behaviour* and was voted one of the most influential women of Great Britain by *Good Housekeeping* magazine. She frequently lectures to both the public and medical profession. She lives in Brighton, Sussex, and has four children and two dogs.

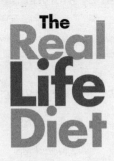

The
Real
Life
Diet

Also by Maryon Stewart

The
Real
Life
Diet

Get the **balance right** and **never** have to **diet again**

Maryon Stewart

PIATKUS

Copyright © 2006 by Maryon Stewart

First published in Great Britain in 2006 by
Piatkus Books Ltd
5 Windmill Street, London W1T 2JA
email: info@piatkus.co.uk

This edition published in 2007

The moral right of the author has been asserted

A catalogue record for this book is available from the British Library

ISBN 978 0 7499 2709 7

Text design by Paul Saunders

This book has been printed on paper manufactured
with respect for the environment using wood from
managed sustainable resources

Typeset by Phoenix Photosetting, Chatham, Kent
http://www.phoenixphotosetting.co.uk
Printed and bound in Great Britain by Clays Ltd, St Ives plc

We are indeed much more than what we eat,
but what we eat can nevertheless help us to be
much more than what we are.

Adelle Davis, the 'first lady' of nutrition

Contents

Acknowledgements

I would never have been able to write this book were it not for my wonderful patients over the last 20 years who have given me the clinical experience and the insight to write a book that has the potential to help millions of other people around the world get back into the driving seat of life. Those who were willing to share their story, setting aside any embarrassment, in the hope of helping others need an additional thank you.

The hundreds of doctors and scientists around the world who have been involved in research into holistic health and obesity must be acknowledged, as many of their publications have been used over the years to develop the Natural Health Advisory Service Programme, which the Real Life Diet is based upon.

I'm truly grateful to two special women, Judy Piatkus and Gill Bailey, for their foresight and persistence in persuading me to keep at it until I got the complete vision for this book, and to Charlotte Howard, my literary agent, for sorting out the housekeeping in her usual professional manner. I am enormously grateful to Jane Garton, my friend and fellow health writer, for her input and for helping to knock the manuscript into shape.

The dedicated team at the Natural Health Advisory Service, past and present, must be acknowledged for their help and support. Special thanks are due to Carys Glaberson for her help with the appendix, Helen Heap for her past help with recipes and to Shirley May for designing the database that makes our case histories accessible.

Introduction

Want to lose weight and tried every diet under the sun? And despite your best efforts the pounds won't budge or just pile back as soon you return to your normal eating patterns. It's hardly surprising. Are you utterly confused about whether to avoid carbs or eat carbs with a low GI? There is so much conflicting data in the media you are entitled to feel bewildered. The simple fact is diets just don't work. Low carb, high protein, no fat ... fad diets abound. And although you may lose weight in the short term it won't stay off. This is endorsed by recent statistics confirming that in the UK some 57 per cent of women and 55 per cent of men are either overweight or obese. Obesity isn't just unsightly; it is linked to serious conditions like prostate, breast and ovarian cancer, and cancers of the womb, kidney, colon, rectum, gall bladder and pancreas, as well as cardiovascular disease and diabetes.

Unscientific or not, it's estimated that, in the Western world, about one-third of women and a quarter of men are on a weight loss diet at some stage, 75 per cent of us are said to be eating fewer carbs and it seems that millions adopt a low carbohydrate diet despite the fact that it has been shown to be harmful to our health in the long term. The only way to seriously maintain weight loss and retain your health is to change your eating habits for life, reduce the serving sizes and get the balance right in your diet, as well as all aspects of your life. Being slim and in good shape isn't just about what you eat and drink, but very much to do with how much stress you have in your life, how physically fit you are and whether you feel loved by others as well as yourself. If life is out of balance then the chances are you won't be sleeping well and your sex drive will have long since diminished. Once you are happy and all aspects of your life are back in balance your weight will stabilise, your skin and hair will glow, and you will be in great shape both mentally and physically. *The Real Life Diet* is aimed at overhauling most aspects of your life, as well as your diet, in order to attain optimum balance. As a result of this diet plan, you will rekindle your zest for life, feel well and be happier with your appearance.

To help you to achieve this balance in your life I have devised a series of questionnaires so you can assess which areas of your life need addressing. It could be that you have low levels of important nutrients, which affect your mood and energy levels as well as your self-esteem, or a lack of focus or something to aim for in your life, not enough exercise, too much stress or just simply an inadequate diet coupled with too much alcohol. It doesn't matter though, for all you have to do is take my simple tests and get going on your own individual Real Life Diet, which I will show you how to tailor to suit your own specific needs based on your test results.

Have a go at answering the following questions and make sure you give honest and spontaneous answers:

How are you doing?

	Yes	No
Do you make excuses in order to avoid having sex?	☐	☐
Can you remember feeling considerably better in the past than you do now?	☐	☐

	Yes	No

Are you more tired than is appropriate for your lifestyle? ☐ ☐

Have you dieted endlessly but feel like you lost the battle? ☐ ☐

Do cravings for food get the better of you? ☐ ☐

Are you confused about which foods to eat in order to stay in good shape? ☐ ☐

Does your skin look less attractive than it used to? ☐ ☐

Are your nails split and brittle? ☐ ☐

Is your hair dull or thin? ☐ ☐

Are you less enthusiastic about starting new projects? ☐ ☐

Has your relationship lost its sparkle? ☐ ☐

Do you often feel stressed? ☐ ☐

Is your libido significantly lower than you would like it to be? ☐ ☐

Do you frequently get irritable and short-tempered? ☐ ☐

Does your life seem full of clutter? ☐ ☐

Do you spend less time looking after yourself than you would ideally like? ☐ ☐

Do you fail to make time to exercise five times a week? ☐ ☐

Is life less enjoyable than you would ideally like? ☐ ☐

Do you rarely have a good laugh? ☐ ☐

Are you aware that you have drifted into the habit of drinking too much alcohol? ☐ ☐

Have you tried to give up smoking without success? ☐ ☐

If you scored more than **one** or **two** Yes answers, then working your way through the Real Life Diet in Part Two of this book will help to restore the balance in your life, leaving you lighter physically, much happier with yourself and in better mental shape too.

Many years of running the Natural Health Advisory Service (NHAS) have led me to realise that when it comes to weight problems the chief culprits are underlying nutritional deficiencies, as a result of either poor eating habits or too many demands on the body, which prevent our brain chemistry from being able to function normally. Too much to do, eating on the run, skipped meals, back-to-back meetings or dashing around after the kids seems to be the order of the day for many. And before you know it your diet is nutritionally deficient in many areas.

The next thing is you start to put on weight, while fatigue, mood swings, skin problems, headaches, aches and pains, food cravings and, in the case of women, hormonal ups and downs and period problems are other common signs that all is not as it should be.

Lurching from one diet to the next, losing weight and then gaining it again does very little for the self-esteem. But it doesn't have to be this way. All you have to do is put your bad habits behind you, and that includes fad diets, and learn how to meet the nutritional needs of your body. The secret is to find the right diet for you and to keep your metabolic rate – the rate at which your body burns up energy – ticking over at an optimum rate with regular exercise. And this is where my Real Life Diet comes in.

To get started on the road to a healthy new slim you just fill in the health questionnaires, which you will find in many of the chapters. Once each one is completed, turn to page 309 where you will find My Real Life Diet and enter your score. In 12 weeks you will need to reassess your score and then calculate the difference to get your Positive Balance Score. This is the difference between the beginning score from all the questionnaires at week 0 and the end score at week 12 – and a measure of your success.

As you go through each chapter make a note of the recommendations you need to follow on your plan and so by the time you have finished Part One of this book your own Real Life Diet will have emerged. Combine these recommendations with Stage 1 of the plan, which begins on page 154, and work your way through the three-stage programme, based on over 20 years of research at the NHAS. It is as simple as that.

And rest assured you won't end up feeling starved and exhausted. Instead you will learn how to meet your body's nutritional needs, which will make you feel better in every aspect of your life. You will feel more alive, more alert, more aware, your sex life will improve, you will feel happier and you will look better too. Your hair and skin will start to glow with a new-found radiance.

Best of all your weight will stabilise naturally and there will be no going back to unwanted bloats and bulges. And there are more benefits too. As soon as you start to become aware of your body's individual nutritional needs everyday niggles such as IBS (irritable bowel syndrome), headaches, cravings, aches and pains, mood swings, anxiety and, for women, premenstrual syndrome, will become things of the past. You also lower your risk of heart disease, diabetes, some cancers, kidney problems, memory loss and osteoporosis.

What are you waiting for? This is your chance to make a plan for yourself that really works; so get started now. . .

Part One

Get Aware

CHAPTER · 1

Assessing your diet

Successfully losing weight and then regaining it time and time again is a recipe for low self-esteem and the last thing you need is yet another weight-loss diet. Instead, you must uncover and really understand the mechanism behind this merry-go-round, so that you can tackle the underlying situation. The Real Life Diet will provide the information that will allow you to find out why you have experienced problems maintaining weight loss in the past and give you the tools necessary to help to address those issues fully. It will give you the opportunity to assess just how overweight you are, as well as discovering what may have contributed to your current relationship with food. It will also challenge you to examine and review where you are at in many other areas of your life so that you can work usefully towards restoring the balance in your life.

Our body automatically sends us in search of food when we are hungry, but some of us eat even when we aren't. Comfort eating, nibbling through boredom or because we are hooked on the flavour and mouth feel of certain foods like chocolate, or simply grazing instead of eating proper meals, are all recipes for disaster. Food is so often regarded as a comfort because many of us were given nice, sweet-tasting food as children as a reward for good behaviour. These days we may reward ourselves for reaching a goal, an achievement or perhaps console ourselves for failing to achieve or losing out emotionally. And we can usually neatly justify it to the point where we make it feel right. But when the habit gets in the way of us looking or feeling our best, or indeed being healthy in the long term, it's time to take stock and find a way to get back in control.

People so often insist that they are eating a healthy diet, but when it comes to recording their daily intake in a diary, horror and disbelief are the two words that spring to mind when I look at their faces.

This may be the first time you have been asked to stop and analyse your diet. Read carefully through the questionnaire below and tick the boxes that most apply to your eating habits. Be absolutely honest, as you won't be fooling anyone except yourself. Once you have finished marking up the questionnaire you can have a read through the results to see how you did. If you do really well you can pat both yourself and your parents on the back, because it is likely that the example you were set at home as a child has rubbed off. If, on the other hand, you don't do so well, don't feel too badly about it because millions of people are in the same boat and you can do something about it.

Is your diet good for you?

Tick the box most relevant to your consumption in each category:

Food	Optimum	Dodgy	Really Bad
Cows' milk (full cream or semi-skimmed, not skimmed)	2 litres or more per week ☐	1–2 litres per week (unless on an exclusion diet and replaced by soya milk – see below) ☐	Less than 1 litre per week (unless on an exclusion diet and replaced by soya milk – see below) ☐
Soya milk (calcium fortified)	2 litres or more per week ☐	1–2 litres per week ☐	Less than 1 litre per week ☐

Food	Optimum	Dodgy	Really Bad
Cheese (full or reduced fat)	125–250 g per week ☐	50–124 g per week ☐	0–49 g per week ☐
Eggs	3–6 per week ☐	1–2 per week ☐	None ☐
Main meal – with protein (animal or vegetarian)	Every day ☐	5 or 6 per week ☐	4 or less per week ☐
Breakfast	Every day ☐	5 or 6 per week ☐	4 or less per week ☐
Fruit, vegetables and salad	5 or more servings per day ☐	3–4 servings per day ☐	2 servings or less per day ☐
Butter	25 g or less per week ☐	Over 25 g but less than 50 g per week ☐	More than 51 g per week ☐
White bread	None ☐	1–2 slices per day ☐	3 or more slices per day ☐
Wholegrain bread	2–3 slices per day ☐	1 slice per day ☐	None – unless you are on a wheat-free diet ☐
Vegetable oil	1 tsp per day ☐	Between 2 tsp and 1 tbsp per day ☐	More than a tbsp per day ☐
Hard margarine	None ☐	Up to 25 g per week ☐	26 g or more per week ☐
Glasses of water	6 or more glasses per day ☐	3–5 glasses per day ☐	Less than 2 glasses per day ☐
Tea and coffee	0–2 mugs per day ☐	3–5 mugs per day ☐	6 mugs or more per day ☐

Food	Optimum	Dodgy	Really Bad
Alcohol	1 drink per day (less than 10 units per week) ☐	8 to 14 drinks per week (11–20 units) ☐	15 drinks (21 units per week or more) ☐
Cola-based drinks (non-diet and diet)	0–1 per week ☐	2–3 per week ☐	4 or more per week ☐
Chocolate bars or equivalent	0–1 bars per week ☐	2–3 bars per week ☐	4 or more per week ☐
Biscuits	0–4 per week ☐	5–14 per week ☐	15 or more per week ☐
Cakes and puddings	0–2 per week ☐	3–5 per week ☐	6 or more per week ☐
Sweets	0–1 per day ☐	2–3 per day ☐	4 or more per day ☐
Teaspoons of sugar added to each tea or coffee	None ☐	½–1 tsp ☐	1 or more ☐
Pizza and white pasta	0–1 servings per week ☐	2–3 servings per week ☐	4 or more servings per week ☐
Packets of crisps	0–1 per week ☐	2–3 per week ☐	4 or more per week ☐
Salt added in cooking or at the table	Never ☐	Occasionally ☐	Regularly ☐
Fish	2 or more servings per week ☐	1 serving per week ☐	Never ☐

Food	Optimum	Dodgy	Really Bad
Lean red meat	3 portions per week ☐	2 or less or more than 5 portions per week ☐	0–1 per week ☐
Sausage, pies and bacon	0–3 times per week ☐	4–5 times per week ☐	6 or more times per week ☐
Takeaways (burger, pizza, Chinese, Indian, fried chicken, fish and chips)	0–1 per week ☐	Twice per week ☐	3 or more per week ☐
Fresh potatoes (not chips)	4 or more times per week ☐	2–3 times per week ☐	1 or less per week ☐
Skip a meal	Never ☐	1–2 per week ☐	3 or more per week ☐

Results

- A score of **25 or above** in the Optimum column means you are doing really well with your diet.

- A score of **18–24** in the Optimum column means that you are not doing too badly, but there is room for improvement.

- If you score **17 or less** in the Optimum column and everything else is in the Dodgy column, you will need to make a real effort to improve your eating habits.

If most of your scores were in the Dodgy and Really Bad columns your diet needs a complete overhaul – Stage 1 of the Real Life Diet beckons! Look on the positive side; because your diet has been so bad, you are likely to experience a great sense of well–being, together with loss of excess weight, once you are through the withdrawal symptoms that can be experienced during Stage 1 of the Diet and consuming much healthier options. Take comfort in the fact that you are not alone and about to gain some amazing knowledge as you go through the Real Life Diet, which will more than make up for anything you haven't learned before.

Write down your score in the notes section of your Real Life Diet on page 309. I want you to repeat this questionnaire again in three months' time and compare your scores.

The benefits of good nutrition

All the evidence indicates that our nutritional state has a major bearing on our future health prospects. Good nutrition has been shown to have all of the following benefits, and probably a great deal more:

- A diet high in fruit and vegetable fibre, low in animal fats and rich in the antioxidant vitamins A, C and E, can reduce the risk of breast cancer by half.

- Eating a diet rich in calcium, magnesium and essential fatty acids, taking regular weight-bearing exercise and by taking supplements of Novogen red clover you can prevent the bone-thinning disease osteoporosis, and reverse it in the early stages.

- A diet rich in B vitamins, in particular B1, B3, B6, B12 and folic acid, vitamin C, essential fatty acids and magnesium, in addition to taking supplements of the same, can help to prevent and treat mental illnesses such as depression, dementia and schizophrenia.

- Consuming a diet rich in essential fatty acids and magnesium, with a low animal fat and salt intake, can help to reduce hypertension (high blood pressure). A study in the USA of 100,000 nurses with high blood pressure discovered that they were magnesium deficient.

- A diet that is particularly rich in essential fatty acids and magnesium can help to unblock clogged arteries and reduce the risk of stroke.

- B vitamins, the antioxidant vitamins A, C and E, the minerals chromium and zinc, and the essential fatty acids and phyto-estrogens, have all been shown to help to control diabetes.

Real life story

Yorkshire businessman **Irvin Green**, 53, who had been battling unsuccessfully with his weight since his childhood, followed the Real Life Diet Plan and is still amazed by the benefits of radically changing his diet and lifestyle.

❛ I had always had a tendency to put weight on since being a chubby child. I can remember trying to lose weight half-heartedly, but socialising for business purposes made it difficult to stick to any weight-loss programme.

The day of reckoning came when I had to watch a video of myself giving a presentation. I was shocked by my appearance. I looked so large I hardly recognised myself. So I decided to do something about it. I talked it through with my partner and we decided to embark on a healthy weight-loss plan together. On the programme we radically changed our eating habits. We gave up junk food completely and alcohol initially, and began eating lots of fruit, vegetables and salads. We also went for vigorous walks with the dogs. Over the months I lost 36 pounds (16 kg) and felt so much better for it, and my partner lost a significant amount of weight as well.

➤

Losing weight and getting fit has made an incredible difference to all aspects of my life, and it was a surprisingly enjoyable and easy way to do it. I have much more energy, my relationships are better and my self-esteem is much higher too. ❞

CHAPTER · **2**

Learning how to interpret 'Bodyspeak'

What is your body telling you?

Now you have completed the questionnaire 'Is your diet good for you?' on pages 10–13 of Chapter 1, you will have a better idea of your probable nutritional health. Amazingly, there are also dozens of physical signs of nutritional deficiency that appear on our skin, show up in the condition of our hair and in the way our nails grow, and affect our digestive systems, but the vast majority of us don't have the knowledge to recognise these deficiencies, let alone correct them.

Plus, there is the question about whether deficiencies really can be corrected only by adjusting our diet. The debate on the pros and cons of taking supplements continues. Some experts say we should, while others maintain we should be able to get all the nutrients necessary for a healthy life from a good diet.

But whichever side you come down on there will always be some people who are deficient in one or more nutrients, or who have special nutritional or medical needs for specific nutrients at certain times in their lives. For example, you may need extra vitamins and minerals if you are getting over an illness, if you are pregnant or are breastfeeding, if you smoke, if you are an athlete or if you often skip meals. You may also need more nutrients as you grow older. You can read more about your specific nutrient requirements through the various life stages in Chapter 3, beginning on page 26.

If you scored 20 or above in the questionnaire on pages 10–13, the chances are your diet is sufficiently high in nutrients to be of benefit. However, if your scores were not so good, you would probably benefit from taking some supplements, especially in the short term, while you make improvements to your diet and allow time for them to take effect. Having low levels of important nutrients will affect your brain chemistry and this may prevent your body from being able to work in an optimum way. This makes it difficult for your metabolic rate to tick over at an optimum level, which may well interfere with your ability to lose weight and maintain the loss. You are also unlikely to feel energised and generally well.

Before you decide whether you need to take supplements and if so which ones to go for, take the test below to help you assess the nutrient levels in your body. Our bodies are good at communicating their deficiencies; it's just that we haven't learned how to interpret the messages, so have a look at the following chart and see how many of the physical signs of vitamin and mineral deficiency are familiar to you.

Are you in good nutritional shape?

Take the test, marking yes or no against each sign or symptom:

Sign or symptoms	Yes	No	What could it indicate?	Action
1. Fatigue	☐	☐	Anaemia Vitamin B or magnesium deficiencies Underactive thyroid	See your doctor for appropriate blood tests (including vitamin B12 if vegan or vegetarian) Consider strong multivitamin and mineral supplement

Sign or symptoms	Yes	No	What could it indicate?	Action
2. Pale appearance	☐	☐	Anaemia – iron or folate deficiency Vitamin B12 deficiency	See your doctor for appropriate blood tests (including vitamin B12 if vegan or vegetarian)
3. Recurrent mouth ulcers or sore, smooth tongue	☐	☐	Iron or folate deficiency Vitamin B12 deficiency	See your doctor for appropriate blood tests (including vitamin B12 if vegan or vegetarian) Consider taking multivitamin and iron supplement
4. Sore, bleeding gums	☐	☐	Vitamin C deficiency	Take 1,000 mg vitamin C with bioflavanoids per day Visit your dental hygienist
5. Excessive cracking and peeling of the lips	☐	☐	Vitamin B2 (riboflavin) deficiency	Consider taking a strong vitamin B preparation
6. Cracking at the corners of the eyes	☐	☐	Vitamins B2 and B6 deficiencies	Consider taking a strong multivitamin and mineral supplement
7. Cracking at the corners of the mouth	☐	☐	Iron and/or mixed vitamin B deficiencies Thrush and eczema	Multivitamin with iron See your doctor if it persists
8. Red, greasy skin at the sides of the nose	☐	☐	Vitamin B2 (riboflavin) and/or vitamin B6 and/or zinc deficiencies	Strong B complex supplement and 15 mg of zinc per day
9. Combination skin	☐	☐	Mixed vitamin B and/or zinc deficiencies	Strong B complex supplement and 15 mg of zinc per day

Sign or symptoms	Yes	No	What could it indicate?	Action
10. Persistent dandruff	☐	☐	Biotin and essential fatty acid deficiencies	Multivitamins, biotin 500 mcg and high strength fish oils Antifungal, tea-tree or tar-based shampoos
11. Eczema	☐	☐	Possible omega-6 essential fatty acid deficiency if excessive dryness	Evening primrose oil 3,000 mg per day See doctor for allergy assessment and infection inspection
12. Red, scaly skin in sun-exposed areas	☐	☐	Vitamin B3 (nicotinamide) deficiency	Strong vitamin B supplement with 100 mg of nicotinamide
13. Acne	☐	☐	Possible zinc deficiency	Zinc supplement 15 mg per day (30 mg if supervised)
14. Psoriasis	☐	☐	Possible mixed vitamin B, zinc and essential fatty acid deficiencies	Strong multivitamin, zinc supplement 15 mg and high strength fish oils Combine with conventional treatment
15. Excessively dry skin	☐	☐	Possible mixed deficiency of essential fatty acid, vitamin A and vitamin E	Multivitamin and mineral supplement with evening primrose oil 2,000 mg and high strength fish oil, plus 400 iu of vitamin E
16. Rough, red, pimply skin on the upper arms and/or thighs	☐	☐	Nothing if mild. If severe, mixed vitamin and essential fatty acid deficiencies	Multivitamin and mineral supplement with evening primrose oil 2,000 mg and high strength fish oil Better diet

Sign or symptoms	Yes	No	What could it indicate?	Action
17. Depression, low libido, anxiety and PMS (for more on these specific conditions, turn to pages 104 and 114)	☐	☐	Possible mixed vitamin B and/or magnesium deficiencies	Magnesium-rich strong multivitamin and mineral supplement with additional magnesium 150–300 mg per day
18. Split, brittle or flattened or upturned nails	☐	☐	Iron deficiency	Iron supplement See your doctor if persistent
19. Ridged nails and white spots on nails	☐	☐	Uncertain significance, possibly iron and zinc	Multivitamin and mineral supplement Better diet
20. Poor hair growth or generalised thinning and loss of hair	☐	☐	Mild iron and vitamin C deficiencies	Take iron and multivitamin supplements and 1,000 mg of vitamin C See your doctor for tests for anaemia, including serum ferritin and thyroid function
21. Loss of sense of taste	☐	☐	Possible zinc deficiency	Zinc 15 mg per day (30 mg if under supervision) See your doctor if it persists
22. Poor vision at night or in the dark	☐	☐	Possible vitamin A (retinol) and/or zinc deficiency	Multivitamin and zinc supplement 15 mg per day (30 mg if under supervision) You **must** see your doctor

Sign or symptoms	Yes	No	What could it indicate?	Action
23. Poor appetite	☐	☐	Zinc, iron and/or mixed vitamin B deficiencies	Multivitamin and multi-mineral supplement See your doctor if you have lost weight
24. Wrinkles	☐	☐	Possible lack of antioxidant (vitamins A, C, E) and the minerals selenium and zinc	Consider taking a good strong multivitamin and mineral preparation
Women only				
25. Heavy periods with flooding or clots	☐	☐	Iron deficiency	See your doctor for blood tests, including serum ferritin Take supplements of iron or iron and multivitamins
26. Painful periods needing painkillers	☐	☐	Possible magnesium deficiency	Consider taking magnesium supplement 150–300 mg per day, evening primrose oil and fish oil
27. Irregular periods	☐	☐	Underweight, low protein diet and excess alcohol	Strong multivitamin preparation Better diet

Results

- If you answered no to **all the questions**, you are a star. The chances are you are in pretty good nutritional shape, and you don't need to take nutritional supplements, unless you particularly want to take a multivitamin and mineral supplement (see page 124), to protect yourself against the potentially harmful effects of the modern environment.

SOME PHYSICAL FEATURES OF VITAMIN AND MINERAL DEFICIENCIES

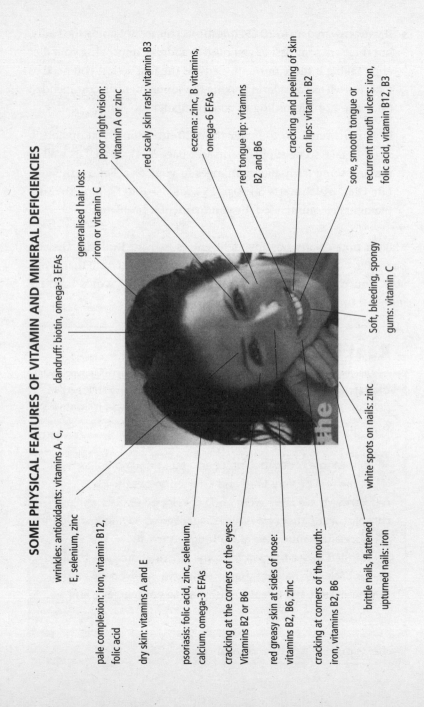

wrinkles: antioxidants: vitamins A, C, E, selenium, zinc

dandruff: biotin, omega-3 EFAs

generalised hair loss: iron or vitamin C

poor night vision: vitamin A or zinc

red scaly skin rash: vitamin B3

eczema: zinc, B vitamins, omega-6 EFAs

red tongue tip: vitamins B2 and B6

cracking and peeling of skin on lips: vitamin B2

sore, smooth tongue or recurrent mouth ulcers: iron, folic acid, vitamin B12, B3

Soft, bleeding, spongy gums: vitamin C

pale complexion: iron, vitamin B12, folic acid

dry skin: vitamins A and E

psoriasis: folic acid, zinc, selenium, calcium, omega-3 EFAs

cracking at the corners of the eyes: Vitamins B2 or B6

red greasy skin at sides of nose: vitamins B2, B6, zinc

cracking at corners of the mouth: iron, vitamins B2, B6

brittle nails, flattened upturned nails: iron

white spots on nails: zinc

- If you answered no to **20–24 questions** you are not doing too badly, but there are some issues you need to address. Improving your diet and making it more nutrient- dense is the first action you need to take, as well as considering taking the supplements recommended (see page 124), according to your particular problems.

- If you answered no to **fewer than 20 questions**, you obviously need to take some supplements (see page 124), as well as well as making some fairly major changes to your diet. Follow the Real Life Diet, which starts on page 154, and consider taking the supplements recommended for your particular problems.

Make a note of any possible deficiencies in your Real Life Diet on page 309. Count up how many ticks you scored and note that down also. You can repeat this test and compare your scores in three months' time.

Real life story

Christine was a 28-year-old actuary, who was very stressed, pressured and out of shape physically. Her symptoms were standing in the way of her progress in life.

❝ Following a root canal infection, I had pneumonia last year. It left me feeling very tired and I started to get thrush regularly. My sex drive went and I developed PMS as well as chronic constipation. I was also diagnosed as having low blood pressure and I put on weight through inactivity.

I decided to see Maryon for some advice about how to get things back into balance. Her programme involved me cutting down on yeast and sweet foods. I had to eat regularly and

➤

take some acidophilus, which helped to calm my gut and the thrush, and a combination of linseeds and magnesium, which worked wonders with the constipation. Plus I took some Optivite (see p 126) and the herb echinacea to help boost my immune system. Within six weeks I felt better. The constipation went and my energy returned. I also began exercising and doing some daily relaxation, which made a big difference. Thrush is no longer an issue and my blood pressure is normal as long as I get enough sleep. My libido has returned, I'm in better physical shape, my weight is back to normal and I feel I have at last got things under control. 〞

CHAPTER · **3**)

Life stages

Different nutrient needs are placed on the body at its different life stages in order that it may continue to function in an optimum way. Usually, as a result of sheer ignorance, increased requirements at crucial times are often not met, which can make it enormously difficult for the body to function at its best. In Chapter 2 we saw how the body is exceptionally good at communicating with us about any deficiencies it may be suffering; it's just that we don't know how to tune in to what the signs really mean. Being in good shape, with a slim, healthy body is all about getting the balance right in your diet as well as in your life.

Learning how to recognise the signs can prevent a lot of misery in the longer term. Whether it's a growth spurt at puberty, peri-menopause in a woman, a mid-life crisis or the 'male menopause', there are very specific changing needs that must be met in order to maintain the body's physical and mental balance. Have a look through the following text relating to the differing life stages and conditions that present themselves at different phases of life, honing in on the ones that are most applicable to your situation in the present, with an eye on where you might be sitting a few years from now.

Stage – Puberty

There are so many rapid changes occurring at the time of puberty it would probably be difficult for the body to keep up even when properly nourished, let alone when firing on two cylinders instead of four, nutritionally speaking. It is therefore little wonder that teenagers often experience extreme mood swings as well as skin problems including heavy bouts of acne. A government survey on young adults in 2000 reported that a staggering 95 per cent of 15–18 year olds had low levels of vitamin B2 in their blood, 54 per cent had low iron intakes, 53 per cent low magnesium, and calcium and zinc were in short supply to the tune of 19 per cent and 10 per cent respectively. The net result of these deficiencies can be dramatic. Having such low levels of so many important nutrients would severely hamper growth and development of everything from brains to bones, and has also been shown to adversely affect concentration and classroom performance as well as behaviour. Poor nutrient levels affect brain chemistry and as a result our self-perception, which may account for the fact that the number of children and young teenagers suffering from eating disorders has doubled in the last few years. They see themselves out of focus and therefore anorexics don't actually see how painfully thin they are and binge eaters don't realise that continually making themselves sick will prevent them from meeting their body's nutritional needs at such a vital time.

To compound the situation further, it has become fashionable for teenagers to drink alcohol, which tends to wash away nutrients, and also to consume inordinate amounts of cola-based and other fizzy drinks, which often impede the absorption of nutrients and can even leach calcium from the bones. Acne, which is usually related to a nutritional imbalance, particularly a lack of the mineral zinc, is at least there for us to see and correct. Many of the other problems created by a lack of nutrients during puberty, like never being able to reach your peak bone mass due to a lack of adequate nutrient intake for various dietary reasons, may well have very serious long-term implications.

Action required

- Ensure a good intake of all nutrients, particularly iron, zinc, calcium and magnesium and essential fatty acids.

- Eat plenty of fresh fruit and vegetable fibre.

- Eat regularly and don't skip meals.

- Try to consume reduced amounts of animal fat, alcohol and cola-based drinks, and refined foods like sweets and crisps.

These measures will all help to improve nutrient levels in the long run and enable the body to work efficiently.

Stage – Being in love

During the initial phase of a new and exciting relationship the body becomes saturated by hormones and brain chemicals that make us feel like we are on Cloud Nine. This is a phase to be treasured in many senses, were it not for the fact that, coupled with the euphoria, appetite often goes out the window. And, while that may be good for the waistline, in the long term it may result in nutritional deficiencies, which can cause mood swings and poor energy levels. So at a time when there is greater physical demand on the body (especially as an hour's active lovemaking uses up at least 150 calories), as well as lots of the mineral zinc being needed for the production of new sperm, it is in our interests to keep ourselves in good nutritional shape.

Action required

- Take multivitamin and mineral supplements if appetite is weak.

- Consider supplements of essential fatty acids and co-enzyme Q10 to help improve stamina and strength.

Stage: Preconception

It is not widely appreciated that both men and women need to pay attention to their preconceptual diet. The health of the sperm as well as that of the unfertilised egg affect the health of the new individual, at birth, in childhood and in the long term, and also have a bearing on the kinds of diseases we end up developing as ageing adults. This has incredibly serious implications, especially when considering that approximately 30 per cent of all pregnancies are unplanned. The upshot for those who are planning their families is that both partners should be undertaking a preconception programme for approximately four months before they begin trying to conceive.

Action required

For both partners

- Take a good strong multivitamin and mineral supplement.

- Keep alcohol to a minimum.

- Avoid contact with chemicals, wherever possible.

- Take regular exercise.

Enjoy a wholesome diet in the form of regular meals and unrefined snacks, like unsalted nuts, dried fruit and cereal bars, together with reduced intakes of refined and fast foods.

Female only

- A daily dose of 400 mcg of folic acid should be taken for four months before pregnancy and for the first three months of the pregnancy. This will help to decrease the chances of having a baby with spina bifida.

- Take B vitamins and essential fatty acids for growth and development of the baby's brain and nervous system.

Stage: Pregnancy

The health prospects of the growing foetus are greatly influenced during pregnancy. Babies who are small for dates are likely to have high blood pressure in later life and, amazingly, even have a different fingerprint pattern to normal-weight babies. Low birth-weight babies are seven times more likely to develop blood sugar problems or develop diabetes than babies whose weight is in the normal range. Impaired lung growth during the developmental stages and early infant life, due to inadequate nutrition and environmental conditions, point to potential abnormal lung function and increased chances of suffering bronchitis, asthma and chronic chest infections.

Action required

Despite the fact that many of us feel incredibly hungry during pregnancy, we don't actually need to eat for two. Our actual requirement for extra calories does not increase significantly in the first six months and it only increases by an additional 10– 20 per cent during the last three months of pregnancy. What does increase is our need for good quality, nutrient-dense foods, which are rich in the following:

- folic acid

- vitamin B12

- essential fatty acids, known to be important for the development of vision and intelligence

- zinc

- iron

- vitamin A, which has been linked to growth

It's important to consume a wholesome diet in the form of regular meals and regular snacks of fresh fruit, unsalted nuts, dried fruit, raw vegetables with dips and home-made cakes and biscuits using fruit, ground almonds and thoroughly cooked eggs, and to avoid drinks containing caffeine and alcohol as these are transferred across the placenta to the growing baby. Plus, take a balanced multivitamin and mineral supplement, together with the specially formulated supplement Mumomega from Equazen (available from high street chemists, health food stores and by mail order from the Natural Health Advisory Service, see page 328).

Stage: Breastfeeding

Nutrient demands on the body during breastfeeding are probably greater than at any other time in a woman's life. Mother Nature attempts to make sure that adequate nutrients go sailing out across the placenta to the growing baby. Despite this, essential fatty acid levels are known to drop to unacceptable levels within a few months following birth; hence breastfeeding mothers need to ensure that they are eating and drinking as often as they feel the need and that their diets are nutrient dense.

Action required

- Eat plenty of wholesome food whenever hunger pangs occur.

- Consume plenty of liquid either in the form of water, watered-down fruit juice, milk, soya milk or herb tea.

- Consider taking a good strong multivitamin and mineral supplement.

- Take approximately 6 capsules of Equazen's Mumomega daily (available from high street chemists, health food stores and by mail order from the Natural Health Advisory Service, see page 328).

Stage: Flagging libido

Good sex not only makes us feel happy and fulfilled, but is also good exercise that helps to keep our bodies toned and our metabolic rate ticking over. When nutrient levels in the body drop below an acceptable level the body goes into what I call 'economy mode'. At this point we manage to continue to perform the basic functions like breathing, eating, existing and sleeping, but commodities like energy, a sense of humour and libido are perceived as being luxuries that cannot be accommodated. Stress in life doesn't help either and nor does an all-encompassing, overburdened work schedule, nor disturbed nights tending the needs of young children. It's all too easy to fall into a trap of neglecting yourself as well as your relationship when life's demands seem to be constantly tugging at you. Libido, or lack of it, is so important to our overall well-being that it merits a chapter to itself, which you will find on page 93.

Action required

- Make time to exercise and rest regularly and pamper yourself with massage, candlelit aromatherapy baths and rich body lotions.

- Consume a wholesome diet.

- Try some of the natural products that have been shown in clinical trials to significantly boost libido, such as horny goat weed or ArginMax (see pages 96 and 97).

Stage: Stressed

More than half the adult population claims to be suffering with stress to some degree. So many of us live life in the 'fast lane', but it inevitably has its drawbacks, and becoming stressed out is one of them. It's all too easy to get overwhelmed by life's pressures and then lose sight of the big picture. A little stress is thought to be good for us, as it keeps us on our toes. However, when stress becomes over-burdening and results in causing us to feel distressed, then it can be extremely bad for both our health and well-being. In this highly pressured situation increased numbers of us keel over from heart attacks or get struck down with irritable bowel syndrome (see page 100). It's not only the high flying executives that are suffering, but so too are exhausted mothers, unemployed and homeless people. And it's not just hype either. A paper published in the *British Medical Journal* confirmed that women who developed breast cancer were far more likely to have experienced bereavement, redundancy, home-lessness, violent crime or family crises within the past five years than their healthy counterparts. A study of Danish bus drivers also showed that those who faced the worst traffic died earlier than their colleagues who drove on country routes.

Action required

- You must leave your working day behind you in order to stand a chance of being able to relax in the evenings. If your stress comes from work, discuss with colleagues how you can make changes, or if you are self-employed you will need to re-evaluate. Try taking some exercise when you finish work, like going for a walk or doing some dancing to your favourite music to help focus your mind on the evening ahead.

- Rekindle your romance on a regular basis – try a candlelit dinner followed by a massage from your partner with some sweet-smelling aromatherapy oil like lavender or geranium.

- Laugh a lot, for research shows that laughter eases stress.

- Try taking a daily supplement of rhodiola, the king of all stress-busting herbs and native herb of Siberia, which has been researched in Russia since the 1930s and has been shown to enhance the systems that regulate stress and help the body main-tain fuel reserves to cope. It is an effective anti-depressant and, as an added bonus, has a reputation as an aphrodisiac, probably due to its ability to lift mood and improve stamina.

Stage: Perimenopause

The perimenopause is the term that defines the five or so years that lead up to the menopause, when oestrogen levels begin to fall and as a result numerous changes begin to occur in a woman's body. Premenstrual syndrome (PMS) may get worse during this phase, and we know that women who suffer with PMS are likely to have low levels of important nutrients including magnesium, which were found, in three separate studies, to be in short supply in between 50–80 per cent of all women. PMS is dealt with in more detail on page 104 of Chapter 10.

Action required

It is vitally important to look after yourself during this phase of your life, particularly ensuring that you are taking in plenty of good nutrients through your diet and the correct supplements to help to redress the balance of both nutrients and oestrogen in your body (see page 124). If you suffer with PMS follow the recommendations outlined on page 104 in order to overcome your symptoms by nourishing the brain chemistry. Keeping yourself in good shape during this stage of your life will pay so many dividends later on.

- Exercise five times each week to the point of breathlessness.

- Cut down your alcohol consumption.

- Concentrate on eating well.

- Try using Arkopharma's Phyto Soya Age Minimising face cream and body lotion (see page 129) to help restore the oestrogen balance in your skin.

Stage: Mid-life crisis/male 'menopause'

Although men are not officially supposed to suffer with a menopause, and indeed they can't exactly, because menopause literally means an end to menstruation, many men do appear to hit an all-time low in their forties or early fifties that definitely seems to be associated with the ageing process. When you stop to consider that just over 100 years ago we weren't living much past 50, the additional years many of us are fortunate enough to be able to potentially enjoy can bring with them added complications, including coping with the ageing process. Just as women have to come to terms with trading youthful looks for wisdom, men have to get to grips with their decreasing prowess, possibly expanding waistline and often thinning locks. While a good percentage of men seem to take these changes in their stride, others get depressed and withdrawn for a while and some even make huge life changes including career moves, altering location and even opting for new and younger partners! Having to cope with so many emotional changes can understandably feel like a crisis. If you are bored with your work life or you have simply had enough of being under pressure, maybe it is time to consider how you could phase yourself into a new and more enjoyable career. While stale relationships can sometimes be resurrected with time, attention and counselling, because of our increased lifespan, more of us seem to be deciding to start new relationships in mid-life. It is perfectly possible to stay in the driving seat following your mid-life re-evaluation, but you have to continue to work at it.

Action required

- Get yourself into good shape nutritionally.

- Keep fit by exercising regularly.

- Take some time out, maybe alone, or with a good friend, to review your life and work out how to welcome the changes.

- If your libido or erectile function has diminished, see Chapter 9.

- If your waistline is heading west, follow the Real Life Diet starting on page 154. Try the supplements glucosamine, the EPA-rich cardiozen (see page 125) and strong multivitamins and minerals to help with developing aches and pains.

Stage: Menopause

The menopause, which signals the end of a woman's fertility, and the action you need to take to overcome the symptoms and emerge in brilliant shape without using hormone replacement therapy, is described in Chapter 10 on page 107.

Stage: Making the most of the extra years

Instead of feeling that life as you knew it is over and that you have now nothing much to look forward to except decline, the years following mid-life can be some of your best if you know how to keep yourself in good shape. It's a time when you no longer have a young family to care for on a daily basis; the chances are you are in a more stable financial position than in years gone by and you have more time to do things that you actually enjoy. So, as long as you are healthy and relatively free from aches and pains, you will be in a good position to enjoy your life to the full. Keeping in good shape is the key. Taking time to meet your changing nutritional needs, exercising regularly as though it's a religious practice, doing a formal session of relaxation daily and having some good old-fashioned goals to achieve in your leisure, will keep you feeling bright eyed and bushy tailed.

Action required

- As your metabolic rate will probably have slowed down by now, in order to prevent gaining weight it is important to consume regular amounts of nutritious wholesome food, but a little less of it. Plan your weekly menu, especially if you are now only cooking for one or two people.

- Eat phytoestrogen rich foods, including soya products and linseeds, to keep hormones in balance and help to prevent heart disease, osteoporosis, diabetes and memory loss. Also consider phytoestrogen supplements.

- Take a daily supplement of Novogen Red Clover, the standardised red clover formulation that will provide 40 mg of isoflavones per day (see page 127).

- Calcium and magnesium supplements help keep your bones strong and muscles working efficiently.

- Essential fatty acids help to protect the faculties and keep the joints flexible and the heart healthy.

- Vitamin D is important for bone strength, if deficient.

- Make sure you eat plenty of oily fish, fruit, salad and vegetables on a regular basis.

- Regular exercise is the key to staying trim and supple.

- A daily session of formal relaxation, including creative visualisation (see pages 84 and 77), will keep you feeling good, for research shows that it can fool your body into feeling that it has accomplished certain activities that it may now be impossible to achieve physically!

Real life story

Simon Haines is a 59-year-old business man from Sussex who spent years yo-yo dieting and never managed to maintain the weight loss.

❝ I have had spates of being overweight all of my life and tried every fad diet going but without success. But after talking to Maryon, and deciding I wanted to make the most of my years, I settled for a healthy eating plan that included a lot of fresh fruit and vegetables and fish, and gave up the foods that turned out to be my downfall.

Not only did I lose weight, I also became much healthier generally. I now manage to control my cravings for sweet and fatty food by eating dried fruit and nuts accompanied by a piece of fresh fruit, or avocados and oily fish such as sardines, which I now know have excellent health benefits.

I only buy healthy food and take no notice of counting calories or carbohydrates, as having attempted to do it years ago, I found it boring, compulsive and counterproductive.

I also walk and swim whenever possible, and I've lost over 30 lb (13 kg) in the last 18 months, which has improved my self-esteem enormously. I started actively socialising again and have found a wonderful partner who makes me feel younger than ever. I'm happier with myself and my life than I can ever remember and am so glad that I have learnt how to control my body. ❞

CHAPTER 4

Food problems and temptations

Are you food sensitive?

Conditions like irritable bowel syndrome (IBS), chronic fatigue and apparent food intolerances or allergies are on the increase in the Western world. Over the years at least 50 per cent of those who attend our clinics are experiencing bowel disturbances, such as constipation, diarrhoea, abdominal wind and bloating. Even larger numbers of people seem to suffer fatigue, headaches and a general lack of well-being. Often these symptoms appear to be related to the diet. It has almost become fashionable to say you have a 'food allergy', but the word 'allergy' simply means altered reaction, and it is often misused by both doctors and their patients.

In our clinics we have discovered that when individuals are in better nutritional shape and no longer consuming a diet full of chemicals and processed foods, their immune function improves and those apparent 'food allergies' often turn out to be transient sensitivities that can be overcome.

Food sensitivity and weight problems

Part of our individuality is determined by the functioning of the immune system. This system produces white cells and antibodies (blood proteins) that help us resist infection. It is able to recognise substances as being either part of the body's metabolism or a 'foreign' substance from outside. Some individuals may become unusually sensitive to these foreign substances and this in turn triggers the 'allergic' reaction. One example is sensitivity to gluten – a protein found in wheat – producing coeliac disease, a condition where the lining of the bowel becomes damaged, making normal absorption of nutrients difficult.

Sometimes, changes in the blood, either in the white cells or in the antibodies, cannot be detected in people who react adversely to foods. In such cases, the term 'food intolerance' is then used. It is becoming increasingly appreciated that while food allergies may be relatively rare, food intolerance may be much more common, and usually produces milder symptoms.

Often when the brain chemistry is adversely affected by a lack of important nutrients the immune system finds it difficult to work efficiently. When our immune system is impaired it can misidentify certain foods and drinks as being 'toxins'. At this point a chemical reaction can occur in the body and as a result fluid floods the cells in an attempt to flush out the identified 'toxin'. Fluid retention and weight gain are common side effects of this phenomenon. In fact, I have seen patients who, once they exclude the 'toxic' foods or drinks, lose up to a stone (6 kg) in the space of a month, simply by passing the redundant fluid as the chemical reaction subsides. Interestingly, a few months down the line, once nutrient levels are back within an optimum range, the previously offending foods or drinks can be reintroduced without any further chemical reaction, and weight levels remain normal. This is a classic example of how getting the nutritional balance right can help us to control our weight.

Foods and allergies

Food allergies are known to play a part in eczema, asthma, nettle rash, rhinitis, swelling of the lips or throat, rheumatoid arthritis and migraine. Food intolerance may aggravate irritable bowel syndrome (IBS), which is estimated to affect at least 20 per cent of men and nearly 25 per cent of women. The sufferer experiences either constipation or diarrhoea, often in association with excessive abdominal bloating and sometimes pains, usually cramp-like and situated either in the middle or lower part of the abdomen. There are no really effective conventional medical treatments for IBS, but it is acknowledged by experts that a change of diet and the introduction of formal relaxation can help to control symptoms in the majority of cases. Research into IBS at Addenbrooke's Hospital in Cambridge, led by Dr John Hunter, revealed the connection between diet and IBS. Surprisingly, one of the commonest foods implicated in IBS was wheat, especially in the form of bran and wholemeal bread. Other common dietary triggers for IBS include milk, cheese, tea, coffee, alcohol and even cigarettes. You will find more on beating IBS in Chapter 10 on page 100.

Migraine headaches can also be triggered by certain foods, as well as stress. The commonest foods to cause a migraine are alcoholic drinks, cheese, pickled foods, chocolate, tea, coffee and foods rich in yeast, such as Marmite and savoury foods or sauces containing yeast extract. If you suffer with migraine, it may be worth noting what foods you have consumed before an attack.

Test your food sensitivity

Think about the following questions and answer Yes or No:

	Yes	No
Do you feel tired after eating?	☐	☐
Do you experience abdominal bloating?	☐	☐

	Yes	No
Do you suffer with wind?	☐	☐
Do you find it incredibly difficult to lose weight?	☐	☐
Are you constipated?	☐	☐
Do you experience diarrhoea?	☐	☐
Do you have tummy aches?	☐	☐
Do you suffer indigestion?	☐	☐
Do you get frequent mouth ulcers?	☐	☐
Do you suffer skin rashes?	☐	☐
Do you have pimples?	☐	☐
Do you get patches of eczema?	☐	☐
Do you suffer with asthma?	☐	☐
Do you get headaches or migraines?	☐	☐
Have you got puffy eyes or a blocked nose?	☐	☐
Do you generally lack energy?	☐	☐
Are you often depressed?	☐	☐
Do you feel on edge and anxious?	☐	☐
Do you experience mood swings?	☐	☐
Do you suffer with rheumatoid arthritis?	☐	☐

Each of the symptoms listed above can be related to food intolerance. If you ticked just **one** symptom from the list, food intolerance or sensitivity is a possibility, **two** ticks and your chances are increasing, and more than **three** ticks means it's likely that your symptoms are food related. Don't forget to enter your score on your Real Life Diet on page 309.

When it comes to detecting food sensitivities there are no hard and fast rules. The most common offenders are grains like wheat and wheat bran, oats, barley and rye, and dairy products including milk, cheese and cream. Stage 1 of the Real Life Diet, which begins on page 154, will give you the opportunity to follow an exclusion diet initially, designed to help you find out whether dietary factors are influencing your well-being and ability to lose weight and remain slim.

Real life story

Bonnie was a 27-year-old journalist, who had come from Australia to work in England. She developed her symptoms once in England and put on 11 lb (5 kg).

❛ I noticed that I was no longer able to control my weight or my moods before my period. I felt very tired and was experiencing bloating and constipation for much of the month. I read about Maryon's work in a magazine and decided to go to see her.

She put me on her Real Life Diet, which involved cutting out all sorts of food including wheat and dairy products initially. In addition I went off to exercise at the gym regularly. The bloating and constipation went almost immediately, and I lost a bit of weight. I no longer felt like sleeping after lunch, which was an added bonus.

Within a few months I had returned to my normal weight and felt so much better for it. I could get my clothes on again and felt so much better about myself. I also noticed that my PMS had gone completely, my concentration was back, and I no longer had any pains or headaches with my period. I

➤

reintroduced dairy products and most of the other grains without any problem.

I can really say I now feel great. I love my diet and my exercise routine, and I feel very much in control of my health. **9**

Addressing your food cravings

Craving food, particularly chocolate, is very common; affecting a staggering 75 per cent of women in the UK to some degree, with 60 per cent admitting that chocolate is their problem. It's not just a female thing. Research shows men are also chocolate cravers. And it's often the cravings getting the better of us that causes us to pile on the pounds and subsequently find it impossible to lose that extra weight.

Interestingly, there is often a physiological reason for cravings. The brain and nervous system require a constant supply of good nutrients in order to function normally but our stressful lives mean that we don't always eat as healthily as we should. We skip meals or eat on the run. As a result our blood-sugar levels drop and we start to crave a glucose fix to give us energy. So what do we do? We grab the nearest bar of chocolate or sweet biscuit, which may give us a quick surge of glucose-fuelled energy but is hardly nutritious. What's more, this quick energy buzz is usually temporary and before too long we are craving something sweet again and so the cycle continues, playing havoc with our waistlines.

The trick is in knowing how to break this cycle, which often develops into a real addiction, and just like alcohol, drugs or smoking, involves a period of withdrawal.

Do food cravings have a hold over you?

Look at the following questions and answer Yes or No:

Yes No

Are you embarrassed about how much chocolate and sweet biscuits you consume? ☐ ☐

Do you graze on chocolate, sweets, biscuits, crisps or similar foods throughout the day? ☐ ☐

Do you make impulse purchases of junk food even when you have resolved not to? ☐ ☐

Do you keep a stash of comfort food at home? ☐ ☐

Do you routinely eat sweet food after meals or in the evening? ☐ ☐

Have you been guilty of eating the children's chocolate? ☐ ☐

Have you bought chocolate as a gift and eaten it yourself rather than giving it? ☐ ☐

If you didn't have chocolate at home, would you sometimes go out especially to buy some? ☐ ☐

Have you had more than three bars of chocolate in the last week? ☐ ☐

Have you had more than three cans of soft drinks in the last week? ☐ ☐

Do you regularly consume ice cream? ☐ ☐

Do you eat biscuits, cake, fruit pies, desserts or other foods containing sugar most days? ☐ ☐

Do you take sugar in your tea or coffee? ☐ ☐

Have you ever eaten chocolate and hidden the wrappers so that no one else would know? ☐ ☐

Yes No

Do you crave salty food like crisps, salted nuts, Marmite or soy sauce? ☐ ☐

Do you feel hooked on certain types of food? ☐ ☐

Do you prefer chocolate to sex? ☐ ☐

If you answered Yes to **three** or more of the questions it's likely that you need to take some action. **Five** ticks means that things are pretty much out of your control and **six** or more gets you the label of Chocoholic! But there is a solution, so don't panic. Don't forget to enter your score on your Real Life Diet on page 309.

How to beat your cravings

A report produced by the Committee on Dietary Reference Values recommends that we cut down our non-milk extrinsic sugars by 50 per cent – this includes any foods or drinks containing sugar. It is not necessarily an ideal recommendation, as it really depends on how much you were eating in the first place. However, it does present an achievable goal that should bring about substantial improvements in both your dental and general health.

Making sure you are getting enough of the right nutrients to keep your blood glucose at optimum levels is key if you want to beat your cravings. The essential nutrients for regulating blood sugar are:

- the B vitamins (necessary for optimum function of the brain and the nervous system)

- magnesium (necessary for normal hormone function)

- the trace element chromium

The B vitamins, magnesium and chromium can be sourced in food, but you have to know where to look for them (see page 299). You may also want to consider taking a specially formulated nutritional supplement that acts as a short-term nutritional prop to regulate blood-sugar levels. For example, Chromium Complex (see page 128) contains B vitamins, magnesium and chromium as well as a little vitamin C and is available through the NHAS Mail Order Service (see page 328).

What and when to eat

When it comes to controlling your cravings, what you eat and when you eat it has a huge part to play. You will be amazed how giving your diet an overhaul and making a few tweaks can help to keep your blood glucose levels on an even keel, which means you are not always longing for your next chocolate fix. As a result you will find the excess pounds will drop off. Here's what to aim for:

- Consume nutritious food little and often to keep blood-sugar levels constant. Eat breakfast, lunch and dinner each day, with a wholesome mid-morning and mid-afternoon snack.

- Eat fresh, home-cooked foods wherever possible.

- Eat foods that are intrinsically sweet like dried fruit, fresh fruit, nuts and seeds.

- Relax while you are eating and enjoy your food.

- Plan your meals and snacks in advance (bearing in mind that calorie requirements are increased by up to 500 calories per day during the premenstrual week for women).

- Always shop for food after you have eaten, not when you are hungry.

- Cut down on tea and coffee. If these are consumed in large amounts, they can cause an increase in the release of insulin. Large amounts of sugar consumed in tea or coffee can also contribute to an unstable blood glucose level. Try Rooibosch, or Redbush, tea, which is a herbal tea look-alike, and coffee substitutes that are available in the health food shops.

- Concentrate on a diet rich in chromium, magnesium and vitamins B and C, including whole grains, chilli, black pepper, chicken, peppers.

- Reduce your intake of alcohol. Apart from the fact that alcohol is high in calories, in excess it can cause liver damage, which can lead to significant hypoglycaemia or low blood sugar. Replacing a meal with two or three gin and tonics, for example, can cause a profound rise and subsequent fall in blood glucose levels, producing all the symptoms of hypoglycaemia.

Get moving

Incorporating regular exercise into your daily life is one factor that can improve the control of blood sugar, speed up your metabolic rate and help you to lose weight, as well as having many other health benefits. Exercise increases the sensitivity of the body's response to insulin, leading to smoother control of blood sugar levels. Ideally, you should be doing at least four sessions of exercise per week to the point of breathlessness.

You will need to set aside some time for planning before you embark on the mission to reclaim your body and your brain. Make notes of all the changes you need to make on your Real Life Diet on page 309. Make a menu plan for the week including snacks, and then go shopping, only buying what is on your list. If you haven't already got one, work out an exercise schedule, even if it is dancing or a workout video at home before the day begins. Also, decide when you are going to steal the time for relaxation, see page 84. It is wise to record how you feel about your physical and mental shape, and your chocolate habits, before you begin, so when you go through the withdrawal symptoms in the first week you will have a reminder to keep you on the straight and narrow.

Real life story

Jackie was suffering with terrible sugar cravings and had put on 2 stone (12.5 kg) in weight as a consequence of over-indulging. I remember her clearly when I first met her in the summer, because her dress wouldn't button at the back and was bulging at the seams. Not surprisingly she was feeling depressed, tense and fairly desperate. I put her on the Real Life Diet, which included taking the supplement Chromium Complex (see page 128). By Christmas she was down to a size 12 from a 16, and her appearance had changed so much that her own brother didn't recognise her when he went to meet her at the station. She was a self-confessed chocoholic, who no longer has any cravings at all. Plus she gave up caffeine and is able to sleep well at night. Her concentration has improved, her PMS has gone, her libido has returned and at her last appointment she took delight in telling me how great she now feels.

Are you addicted?

When our lives get out of balance it is all too easy to use stimulants or comfort foods and drinks as a prop to get us through the day. So if you can't get through the day without a cigarette, a cup of coffee or a glass of wine or cola the chances are you could be addicted, heading towards addiction or at least getting into bad habits. It's time to break the habit before it starts to affect your health and well-being. Comforters such as alcohol and sweet food often cause us to gain weight because of their high calorie content, and so it becomes a vicious circle.

A little bit of what you fancy may do you good but if the word 'little' no longer applies to your lifestyle patterns you could be setting yourself up for all kinds of problems. If you feel you've got an addictive personality now's the time to take stock. Have you ever thought why you reach for that cigarette or glass of wine? It could be a sign that you are looking for an external solution to some problem that is going on inside, which needs addressing.

Although you can't change your personality you can learn to recognise an addictive streak and take steps to keep it in check. Taking the test that follows will help you to decide whether you have an addictive nature; it will allow you to identify any problem areas and help you decide on the best action to take.

Do you have addictive tendencies?

Look at the following questions and answer Yes or No:

Yes No

Caffeine

Do you find it hard to get going if you don't have coffee or tea first thing in the morning? ☐ ☐

Do you get headaches if you don't have your caffeine fix? ☐ ☐

Does a meal feel incomplete without a cup of coffee? ☐ ☐

Does your energy level slump mid-afternoon without caffeine? ☐ ☐

Do you crave chocolate if there is none available? ☐ ☐

Do you choose cola-based drinks over fruit juice or water? ☐ ☐

Do you find it hard to sleep or do you feel restless in the night? ☐ ☐

Alcohol

Do you have more than two drinks a day (for women)/three drinks a day (for men)? ☐ ☐

Do you never have a day in the week without alcohol? ☐ ☐

Do you drink alcohol with every evening meal? ☐ ☐

Yes No

Do you drink alcohol to make yourself feel better? ☐ ☐

Do you drown your sorrows regularly with alcohol? ☐ ☐

Do you rely on alcohol to boost your confidence? ☐ ☐

Do you feel agitated if alcohol isn't available? ☐ ☐

Smoking

Do you light a cigarette when you feel stressed? ☐ ☐

Do you reach for a cigarette when you feel emotionally
vulnerable? ☐ ☐

Do you smoke to stimulate your thought processes? ☐ ☐

Do you have a cigarette when you wake up in the morning? ☐ ☐

Do you smoke after sex? ☐ ☐

Do you get withdrawal symptoms if you don't have a cigarette? ☐ ☐

Do you have to have a cigarette every time you have an alcoholic
drink? ☐ ☐

If you answered Yes to **any** of the questions in the three sections above it is likely that you have become dependent. Now turn to your Real Life Diet on page 309 to enter your scores.

Giving up cigarettes, cutting down on alcohol and forgoing your cola or caffeine fix isn't easy for anyone. The first steps involve taking a long, hard look at how your addictive tendencies could be affecting your health and well-being, and listening to other people's concerns, as they may be able to help. You also need to challenge any addictive thought patterns, such as it's OK to do this just this once . . . or I'll start giving up tomorrow . . . It may also help to try and address the need behind the cravings, whether it's really craving more emotional security or greater self-esteem.

Once you've got a better insight into your addictive tendencies, read on to find out how to face up to them and kick them once and for all.

Caffeine

You just have to look at all the coffee bars springing up in the high street to see why it has never been so easy to get hooked on caffeine. And it's not just coffee and tea that contain caffeine. Chocolate, chocolate drinks, cola, cola-based drinks, Lucozade, Lemsips, some painkillers and drinks like Red Bull, Red Kick and Virgin Energy are also laced with caffeine.

Although small amounts of caffeine can make you more alert and enhance your concentration, in excess it quickly becomes an unhealthy substance. It can make you tense, nervous and anxious. It may also trigger a rapid pulse and palpitations, and has been linked to heart disease, high blood pressure and even infertility, as well as aggravating breast tenderness in women.

Caffeine is not an easy substance to give up as total withdrawal can give you headaches, tremors, nausea and diarrhoea. Cutting down gradually is the best way forward and, if you can, you should plan your first 'without-days' over a weekend so you can take it easy if withdrawal symptoms hit you hard.

Coffee

Breaking the habit

- Reduce your intake gradually over a couple of weeks.

- Allow yourself no more than two cups of decaffeinated coffee a day.

- Try coffee alternatives such as barley cup, dandelion coffee or 'no caff' drinks, all of which are available from health food shops.

- If you like filter coffee you can carry on using your filter but with decaff versions or you could try roasted dandelion root, also available from health food shops. All you have to do is grind it and put it through the filter, as you would with ground coffee.

Tea

You may find it hard to imagine a day without a cuppa but the truth is it's full of caffeine and another nasty substance called tannin, which inhibits the absorption of nutrients, especially zinc and iron. You can expect the same withdrawal symptoms as with coffee and you may also become constipated without tea, so it's best to ditch teatime slowly.

Breaking the habit

- Follow the same advice as for coffee.

- Herbal teas are good alternatives, as all are free of caffeine and tannin. Lemon and ginger, fennel and mixed berry are firm favourites. Rooibosch Eleven O'clock tea is another one to try. It takes a while to get used to, but once you do you may find you prefer it to ordinary tea.

Caffeinated fizzy drinks

They may be refreshing, stimulating and, if we are to believe the ad men, good for our image. But caffeinated fizzy drinks are also full of sugar (approximately eight teaspoons per can of cola), not to mention all the other chemical additives. Diet versions may not have the sugar but their chemical additive count is sky high. To help you give up, follow the weaning advice as for coffee, but be prepared as you may start to experience similar withdrawal symptoms such as headaches and nausea.

Breaking the habit

- Follow the same advice as for coffee.

- Try some of the healthier fizzy drinks you may find on supermarket shelves, such as Appletize, Amé and Irish Spring. Check out the labels for caffeine and added sugars and chemicals.

- Make your own fizzy drinks by diluting fruit juice with some fizzy water.

Alcohol

We don't need to be reminded that too much alcohol is bad for health and our waistlines as it has such a high calorie content. A couple of glasses of wine may actually do you some good, but overindulge and you are laying yourself open for all sorts of medical problems. For a start, alcohol knocks most nutrients sideways and over the years can destroy body tissue. It can also cause or contribute to a host of conditions, including cardiovascular disease, digestive disorders, liver disease, cancer, brain degeneration, miscarriages and osteoporosis, to name just a few.

If you feel you could be drinking too much it is important to seek help before things get out of hand. As a guide we should all try to keep within the government's recommended limits, which are no more than 14 units a week for women and 21 for men. One unit is equivalent to either an average glass of wine or a pub measure of spirit or half a pint of either lager or beer.

Breaking the habit

- Have at least two alcohol-free days a week.

- Alternate alcoholic drinks with soft drinks or water.

- Don't drink more than one unit an hour.

- If you are drinking, set yourself a maximum limit of 3–4 units and stick to it.

- Stick to pub measures of spirits and dilute them well with plenty of mixers.

- Avoid binge drinking (this means more than 8 units in a session).

Cigarettes

Despite national targets to reduce the number of smokers, recent research announced that vast numbers of children are likely to become smokers because they possess addictive genes. And regardless of the fact that there have been repeated government health warnings and awareness campaigns an amazing 26 per cent of us still smoke. But we do so at our peril. There is endless research to show that smoking is the UK's single greatest cause of preventable illness and early death. Although smoking doesn't cause us to gain weight, and in fact smokers often miss meals because cigarettes curb their appetite, we know that smokers tend to drink more alcohol and often choose less nutritious foods that are high in calories.

Tobacco use kills around 106,000 people in the UK every year, more than 300, or a plane load of people, every day – around 20 per cent of all deaths. It also causes a wide range of illnesses including various cancers (lung cancer is the most significant), respiratory diseases and heart disease.

Tobacco contains more than 4,000 chemicals, 43 of which are proven carcinogens, including acetone, ammonia, arsenic, DDT, cadmium and hydrogen cyanide, as well as tar and carbon monoxide. It also reduces elasticity of skin, causing premature ageing.

As a smoker, the single, most important thing you can do for your health is to give up smoking. It won't be easy but within just three months circulation improves, lung function increases by up to 40 per cent and you will find it easier to exercise. Coughing, wheeziness and shortness of breath will also improve. Your skin will start to glow and food will taste that much sharper. As an added bonus you will no longer smell of stale smoke.

Breaking the habit

- Pick a quit date. Tell friends, family, workmates and anyone who can support you when you are going to give up.

- Establish new habits. Before you give up, get into some new healthy habits to keep you busy and distract you. Build in rewards too – save the money you would have spent on cigarettes for a holiday or other treat.

- Get active. Smokers who exercise are more likely to succeed in giving up and less likely to put on weight when they stop.

- Change the way you think. Keep reminding yourself why you want to stop and the benefits of giving up (it may help to write your reasons on a card to carry round with you). Take it a day at a time.

- Plan the first week. Remember that the early days are usually the most difficult. Try to avoid places and people you associate with smoking. Steer clear of pubs, clubs and other places with smoky atmospheres.

- Beat the cravings. If you feel the urge to light up, take a few long, slow breaths, drink a glass of water, use stop smoking aids, go for a walk, see a friend or watch a favourite video. Remember, cravings do pass.

- Stick to it. If you give in and have a cigarette try to work out why and use the experience to help you try again. Most successful quitters have stopped for good only after trying several times. There are 12 million people (around a quarter of all adults) in the UK who have quit. You can join them.

- Rather than using nicotine replacement, which maintains the dependency to nicotine, contact EasyStop (see page 327), who run a successful programme combining counselling, aversion therapy and hypnotism. They help you to examine the reasons why you smoke and establish new habit patterns.

Real life story

Susie was a 24-year-old primary school teacher, who had put on weight and needed help for her severe panic attacks and depression.

❛ I felt fat and depressed and had begun experiencing waves of panic, to the point where I couldn't go into work. I tried, but the panics were so severe that I couldn't get past the door. I had just finished a period at the time, but I didn't connect it. I was also smoking between 30 and 40 cigarettes a day.

After reading one of Maryon's books, I decided to go and see her. She designed a new diet for me, recommended a selection of supplements to help with my symptoms and said I should take regular exercise.

By my first follow-up appointment, a month later, I was feeling happier and less anxious. I cut down my smoking as well as chocolate, cakes and sweets. By the next appointment I was able to hold an assembly for 400 children without panicking, which I felt was a real achievement.

Following Maryon's Real Life Diet, I have now lost a stone without trying and am back to feeling good and in control of my life. So many people have commented about how different I look, and I know how different I feel. I really look forward to work now. ❜

Tips to keep you off the hook

- It can be hard to go it alone. Ask your friends and family for support.

- Think about how much you stand to gain by breaking your addictive cycle.

- Write down all the reasons for your decision to give up and refer to it when the going gets tough.

- Be aware of what you turn to when feeling low and ring the changes by doing something different.

- Learn to spot the warning signs that your cravings could be about to get the better of you. Forewarned is forearmed.

- If you do give in, don't beat yourself up. Just resolve to try again.

- Try to build up your coping skills and problem-solving abilities so you don't have to resort to quick fixes if things start to go wrong.

CHAPTER 5

How fit are you?

The first step in assessing how fit you are is to take a look at how much you are eating and whether or not you are overweight. Then we will go on to look at your lifestyle and how much exercise you do.

Are you eating too much?

Recent government figures show that as a nation we are fatter than ever before and this means a good proportion of us are eating more than is good for our health. According to a survey carried out by the Department of Health in 2003, which has only just come to light under the Freedom of Information Act, more than eight million Britons are now categorised as clinically obese, which puts them at risk of chronic illnesses including heart disease and diabetes.

The survey found that one-quarter of all adults are dangerously overweight and that there has been a 75 per cent increase in obesity in the UK during the past ten years, with the number of dangerously fat women increasing by 50 per cent and fat men by almost 75 per cent. And these figures are replicated throughout much of the Western world.

How did we get like this? Lack of exercise and unhealthy habits are partly responsible, but the main culprit is diet. We are simply eating far more calories than ever before and the body stores excess calories as fat. We also tend to consume more fat, which contains more calories per gram than any other food, expanding our waist-lines even further.

You may well wonder how these trends have come about when millions of us start weight-loss diets each year. But, as we know, often from experience, most diets simply don't work. We may lose the pounds in the short term but nine times out of ten the weight soon comes back once we return to normal patterns of eating and so begins the familiar pattern of yo-yo dieting. The only way to lose weight and keep it off is to follow a balanced eating plan as described in Part Two of this book – Maryon's Real Life Diet in Action.

The BMI test

The words 'fat' and 'overweight' are part of our everyday language, but the term obese isn't so widely understood. If you are classified as obese this means that you are extremely overweight – to a measur-able degree. The following equation will allow you to assess your Body Mass Index (BMI) and check to see whether you are overweight and, if so, to what degree. The grades are divided up into five sec-tions, –1, 0, 1, 2 and 3. These are grades based on weight and height that are taken from the formula originally devised by a Belgian sci-entist, Quetelet. Quetelet's Index, which is now more usually known as BMI, is widely used in the assessment of obesity. The formula is derived by multiplying your height in metres by itself and then dividing your weight in kilograms by this figure:

$$BMI = \frac{weight\ in\ kilograms}{height\ in\ metres^2}$$

The categories are as follows:

-1: Score less than 20

0:   Score 20–25

1:   Score 25–30

2:   Score 30–40

3:   Score greater than 40

If your grade is –1, you are underweight.

Normal or ideal weight is grade 0.

Grade 1 is overweight, usually between 10 and 20 per cent above the ideal weight.

Grades 2 and 3 are regarded as obese – more than 20 per cent above the ideal weight.

Grade 2 and especially grade 3 obesity carry the greatest health risks. An adult with a BMI of 40 has three times the risk of dying in a year than someone whose weight is ideal. An individual with a BMI of 35 has approximately twice the death rate of his or her grade 0 counterpart. So, it's not just a nice idea to shed those additional pounds permanently, it could be a matter of life or death.

For the majority who are just slightly overweight, at grade 1, the major reasons for dieting are cosmetic and to increase well-being. Many of us feel better psychologically when that spare tyre has been whittled away, and if the diet is combined with an exercise programme, there can be a very real improvement in feelings of overall fitness. Medically, there is little change in factors such as blood pressure and risk of heart disease, though there could be a moderate fall in blood cholesterol level if this is high at the start of the diet.

For those with grade 2 or 3 obesity, the potential benefits of losing weight are very real, and the psychological effects of a successful weight-loss programme can be dramatic. For example, normal employment may be very difficult for those who are grossly over-weight, at grade 3 obesity.

People with grade 2 or 3 obesity do have a shorter life expectancy, and an increased risk of many illnesses, including diabetes, high blood pressure, heart disease, osteoarthritis, gout, gallstones, reduc-tion in exercise tolerance/level of fitness and depression. Medical problems may be more difficult to treat in those who are obese. Gastrointestinal disorders, including indigestion, heartburn and constipation, may not be so easy to assess and the survival rate of an obese woman with breast cancer is lower than her slim counterpart.

Those who manage to return to normal or near-normal weight will stand a good chance of returning to a normal life expectancy and a reduction in their risk of medical problems associated with obesity, and certain problems including arthritis, gout, blood pres-sure, diabetes or blood cholesterol levels may be dramatically improved within a few months.

Metabolic syndrome

We know that being obese wrecks self-esteem and increases our risk of developing certain illnesses, but many people don't know that where you store your excess fat is also important. You may hate being blessed with large hips that cause you to be a pear shape, but this is actually better for your health than being apple shaped. Apple shapes tend to store fat round the middle. Being overweight as well means that you are twice as likely to develop heart disease, especially if this runs in your family, as it is thought to be related to the inherited, metabolic ways in which you handle dietary fats and carbohydrates.

Metabolic syndrome, which according to the British Nutrition Foundation is a public health time bomb, is a condition in which the body becomes resistant to the effects of the hormone insulin and, as a result, increases the risk of developing heart disease and stroke. As many as one in five adults in some Western countries are victims, and it can result in premature death. Metabolic syndrome is either the result of inherited genes, or of diet and lifestyle factors, such as eating excessive amounts of sugar and refined carbo-hydrates, together with little or no exercise, which also increases the chances of becoming diabetic.

Body weight plays an important role in the development of this syndrome and with obesity spiralling out of control the problem is only set to get worse. When too many foods that raise blood sugar levels are eaten, more insulin is secreted to help push the excess glu-cose into fat cells for storage as body fat. This encourages the body to produce the classic apple shape. When body cells become in-creasingly insensitive to the effects of insulin, the pancreas is forced to produce increasing amounts of insulin to help maintain normal blood-glucose levels. People with metabolic syndrome are basically overdosing on glucose and insulin and as a result develop a number of symptoms, including difficulty losing weight, tiredness and sugar cravings. Those with metabolic syndrome also tend to develop high blood pressure, raised LDL-cholesterol and a reduced ability to han-dle glucose. LDLs are low density lipoproteins and are designed to transport cholesterol around the body. However, too many LDLs can damage the arteries and place you at greater risk of heart disease.

Apple or pear shaped?

To work out if you are apple shaped, measure your waist and hips using a non-stretchable tape measure. Divide your waist measure-ment by your hip measurement to get your waist/hip ratio. For example, if your waist is 88 cm (34½ in), and your hips are 100 cm (39 in), then your waist/hip ratio is 88/100 = 0.88. A waist/hip ratio greater than 0.85 is apple shaped for women; while a ratio greater than 0.95 is apple shaped for males.

In fact, waist size alone is also a good indicator of health. Men with a waist size of more than 94 cm (37 in), or 80 cm (31½ in) for women, are most at risk of developing weight-related health problems, such as shortness of breath, high blood pressure, high cholesterol levels and diabetes, than those with slimmer waistlines. If your waist size is greater than 102 cm (40 in) for men or 88 cm (34½ in) for women, the likelihood of having metabolic syndrome is very high.

What you can do if you are obese

When it comes to dealing with obesity the bottom line is to eat less and exercise more. If you suspect you could be one of the obese crowd, here are some ideas to kick-start your healthier lifestyle before turning to the Real Life Diet in Part Two of this book, which begins on page 154.

- Your first port of call if you are grade 2 or 3 obese should always be your doctor to check whether your weight problem is due to any medical condition. If tests indicate that you have an underactive thyroid or sluggish metabolism, it may be worth investigating some appropriate complementary therapies as well as any medication you may be prescribed by your doctor. An acupuncturist would be my first port of call, as unblocking the energy channels can help you back to optimum metabolism, but always check first with your doctor before undergoing any therapies.

- Eat regularly, at least three meals a day, preferably with two small snacks in between.

- Never miss meals: irregular eating leads to less healthy weight loss and increased feelings of hunger.

- Eat from a small plate, not a large one. A well-stocked medium-sized lunch or breakfast plate looks more satisfying than a large dinner plate only half filled.

- Chew your food well and savour each mouthful. Try not to hurry your meals.

- Eat fresh foods whenever possible. If at all possible, prepare one meal at a time. If this is not practical, try cooking a chicken, for example, to eat cold over several days.

- Grill rather than fry food to keep your fat consumption low and to preserve the nutrients.

- Do at least four sessions of exercise to the point of breathlessness per week, which will help to speed up your metabolic rate (the amount of energy you produce) and as a result burn the fat off! But if you haven't been exercising regularly for some time, take it easy to begin with (see page 67).

- Consider spending a week at a health retreat to get yourself started – perhaps as part of your annual holiday. There's nothing like having the appropriate food handed to you on a plate, and spending your time being pampered will undoubtedly help you to focus on a new sense of well-being.

- If you have tried endless diets without success and feel you may have a psychological block about losing your weight, ask your doctor about the possibility of having some counselling.

Real life story

South African **Paul Curtis** is a 55-year-old ex-advertising creative director, turned pub owner and writer/publisher, who had been happily overweight for many years, but the problem became so much worse when he spent his days eating and drinking as the landlord of a gastro-pub. The discovery seven years ago that he had adult-onset diabetes shocked him into a radical lifestyle overhaul as he realised that his diet and lifestyle had contributed to the situation.

❝ A sustained diet of junk food, a love of red wine and a lack of exercise saw my weight almost double from what it had been when I was 25.

The ridiculous thing was I was actually quite happy with the way I was, although my wife was always putting me on a variety of diets, with dire warnings that unless I lost weight

➤

and stopped smoking – I was a 60-a-day man – I would ruin my health. But I didn't see myself as fat and I was never sick so what was the point in giving up everything I enjoyed?

The wake-up call came when I began to have problems with my eyesight and was constantly thirsty. After a series of tests my doctor told me that my blood sugar count was astronomical, my blood pressure was through the roof and unless I changed my lifestyle I could drop dead at any time.

The doctor referred me to the professionals at the Centre for Diabetes in Johannesburg and my life changed. I heard about Maryon's programme and followed a strict diet and regular exercise regime. My eyesight slowly returned to normal, and the weight dropped off me. I can't say that it was easy at first but it's amazing how the threat of one's imminent demise can spur one on! I am now literally a shadow of my former self and feel so much better for it. **9**

Measure your fitness level

Getting fit and staying fit through exercise is essential to a long and healthy life, and a vital aid to losing weight and keeping the excess weight off in the long term. Not only is exercise necessary for the optimum function, structure and preservation of muscles, joints, bones and heart, but it also does wonders for your mood and hormones, and can send energy levels soaring. In addition it boosts circulation, keeps your skin looking healthy and helps to burn calories. If you do an hour's vigorous exercise instead of sitting in a chair you could burn up to 200 calories, which otherwise may have gone on to your waistline. It has long been known that men tend to burn calories more easily as they have a higher muscle to fat ratio. So, if you are female and if weight loss has been difficult in the past, increasing your muscle mass through exercise will allow you to lose weight with less difficulty.

As in every area of your lifestyle, when it comes to exercise, balance is key. It is all very well encouraging people to exercise to the point of breathlessness but you need to build up stamina before attempting to do this for any length of time. If you start off exercising too vigorously you risk ending up feeling achy, tired and disappointed. On the other hand, if you don't exercise hard enough to stimulate your limb and heart muscles you might as well not have bothered. If you haven't exercised for a long time or are receiving medical treatment it is best to check with your doctor before embarking on a vigorous exercise regime.

Unless you are an established exerciser, answer the following questions to check your current of fitness before embarking on an exercise plan.

	Yes	No
Are you currently doing no exercise?	☐	☐
Are you currently doing some exercise occasionally?	☐	☐
Do you exercise more than three times a week for more than 30 minutes at a time?	☐	☐
Do you get puffed easily?	☐	☐
Can you run up and down stairs without panting?	☐	☐

Which of the following best describes you?

Very unfit	☐
Moderately unfit	☐
Not as fit as you should be	☐
Moderately fit	☐
Fit	☐
In excellent physical condition	☐

Unless you are exercising regularly and feel comfortable doing so, consider that there is room for improvement. And even if you are fit, you need to bear in mind that you may need to work harder to stay fit and keep your metabolic rate ticking over at an optimum rate as you get older. Read the section below that is applicable to your current position.

If you are very overweight and unfit

- You should check with your GP before starting on a fitness regime. Then you can start exercising gently for 5–10 minutes a day and gradually build up the amount over a month.

- Walking and swimming are good stamina-building exercises.

If you are moderately overweight and not as fit as you should be

- You should start exercising gently, perhaps by going for a walk each day for at least half an hour. Gradually increase your pace to the point where you are walking briskly and you can feel your heart pumping away efficiently. You should be able to carry on a conversation while exercising. If you can't you are could be over-doing it and should relax your pace.

If you are mildly overweight and exercise occasionally

- If you reckon you are a little overweight for your height and could do more exercise than you do, you need to follow an improver's programme. This means stepping up your pace gradually and increasing the number of times you exercise a week.

- Swimming or aqua fit classes will get your muscles working without putting you at risk of post-exercise aches and pains.

If you are overweight but fit

- If you are on the heavy side but exercise at least four times a week, you should carry on with your routine, gradually increasing your pace and maybe adding another session. Continue to stick to a balanced eating plan.

Real life story

Caroline was 18 years old when I first saw her. She was pretty overweight and was suffering with endometriosis, a condition where the lining of the womb grows around other organs in the abdominal cavity.

❜ I had been travelling in Peru for six months and had put on over 2 stone (12.5 kg) in weight. I had previously been diagnosed with endometriosis, which was very painful, especially at period time. My mother suggested I went to see Maryon because of the pains and the weight gain.

I followed Maryon's special diet plan, and took the supplements she recommended. In addition I decided to give up red meat and eat more fish. I also took up regular exercise, which I now know is energising and helps to maintain the weight I lost.

At first I felt worse, but gradually I started to get some real balance into my life. I have lost over 2 stone and feel good. I never binge or eat for comfort any more, and I discovered that I only get bloated if I eat wheat. I still exercise regularly and follow the diet as it makes me feel so much better on every level. ❜

Which exercise?

The secret to sticking to any exercise programme is to choose an activity that you enjoy and one that you are physically capable of. That way you are more likely to stay motivated and look forward to doing it each day. There is little point in arranging to play squash if you hate the game or promising yourself you will go for a jog each day if you loathe running.

Remember that the aim of your activity is to get to the point of breathlessness. This type of exercise, known as aerobic exercise, stimulates the large groups of muscles in your body, getting them to contract rhythmically. Over time these muscles, including the heart, which is a muscular organ, become more efficient. And once you have achieved improved cardiac function you will start to feel better physically and mentally – instead of feeling sluggish you will feel energised and happy.

It is also a good idea to vary the type of exercise you do on different days of the week to stave off boredom. Good aerobic options include running, power walking, cycling, swimming, cardiovascular machines at the gym, tennis, squash, badminton, dancing, roller-blading, hockey, football, rowing, rope skipping or an aerobics-based exercise class. Alternatively you can just stretch and dance to your favourite music. I tune in and work out to Planet Rock on my digital radio before the day begins, and I swear I feel 20 years younger as a result. If you haven't got an established exercise routine I recommend you give it a try.

Try to fit some exercise into your routine on a daily basis and chart the amount you do each day on your charts in the diary section. If you are concerned you may be not be able to stick to an exercise routine it may help if you plan out your week's activity in advance in your diary or on a wall chart. It can also help to exercise with a friend. It's more fun, feels less like a chore and you can catch up on gossip at the same time. You can also motivate each other – you are less likely to cancel your regular workout if you feel you are letting the other person down.

Keep the benefits of exercise uppermost in your mind until your regime is firmly established. When you have reached your goal of doing four or five sessions of exercise a week, work to maintain it but don't exceed it on a regular basis. Believe it or not, too much exercise can be bad for you, putting a strain on your joints and bones.

After each workout really tap into how you are feeling. Because exercise encourages your body to release endorphins, the body's own feel-good hormones, you will feel elated, full of energy and proud of yourself. Hold on to that thought and next time you start to hesitate over whether to work out or not remind yourself how good it makes you feel.

Watch points

- If you are not exercising in a class, remember to warm up and warm down before and after every exercise routine
- Warm up slowly for the first few moments
- Continue until you reach the point of breathlessness – this is the signal to start the cool-down process
- Take a few minutes to cool down gradually rather than stopping vigorous exercise suddenly

Ten ways to sneak fitness into your life

1. Walk around while talking on the phone to friends.

2. Don't use lifts; always use the stairs.

3. Instead of e-mailing colleagues, go to their desks and talk to them.

4. Go for a walk round the block in your lunch hour.

5. Go to the disco instead of the pub and dance yourself fit.

6. Get rid of the remote control and get up to switch TV channels instead of channel hopping from the sofa.

7. Leave the car behind and walk or run to the shops for the newspaper.

8. Put some real effort into the housework.

9. Arrange to meet a mate and walk to the football match instead of having a pint in the pub beforehand.

10. Take up an active hobby that you enjoy such as salsa, t'ai chi, or five-a-side football.

If you would like to check out just how many calories you can burn by keeping fit look at the following website http://www.healthyweightforum.org/eng/calorie-calculator.asp?action=submit

CHAPTER 6

Learning to love yourself

According to the song, learning to love yourself is the greatest gift of all, but it isn't something that comes naturally to most people. People who can't find a multitude of things wrong with themselves are in the minority. You know the old story – your hair is the wrong colour, or it's curly instead of straight or vice versa. Your nose is too long, your eyes too small and your figure is completely the wrong shape. You haven't got as much character as your friends and you're not as clever and so it goes on. But unless you like yourself you don't stand much of a chance of getting your body into really good shape. Show me someone who is happy with their life and their shape and I pretty much guarantee that they have good self-esteem and like who they are. And you will find, on the Real Life Diet, that as each month passes your weight reduces and you begin to like your reflection in the mirror, you will automatically begin to feel much better about yourself.

The truth is that no one is perfect, and many of us will probably never be entirely satisfied with our lot, but we can get close to it. However, while there is always room for improvement, it is important we recognise the good things about ourselves that make us who we are. Find out if you love yourself enough and if you don't, discover what to do get you back on the self-love track. Answer Yes or No to the following questions:

Do you love yourself?

	Yes	No
Do you always think everyone is better looking than you?	☐	☐
Do you dislike your shape?	☐	☐
Do you think you are too fat?	☐	☐
Do you think you are too thin?	☐	☐
Do you avoid looking at yourself in the mirror?	☐	☐
Are you embarrassed to undress in front of others?	☐	☐
Do you shy away from wearing figure-hugging clothes?	☐	☐
Do you skip meals in order to lose weight?	☐	☐
Are you constantly on a diet?	☐	☐
Do you ever make yourself sick after eating?	☐	☐
Do you always concentrate on your bad points rather than your good points?	☐	☐
Do you take no pride in your appearance?	☐	☐
Are you embarrassed to make love with the lights on?	☐	☐
Do you always think your partner is looking at others?	☐	☐
Do you tend to dwell on the failures in your life rather than all the good things that have happened?	☐	☐
Do you smoke or drink alcohol to make you feel better about yourself?	☐	☐
Do you often doubt your ability to succeed?	☐	☐

Yes No

Are you afraid to ask questions in public for fear that you will
be laughed at? ☐ ☐

Do you wish you were someone else? ☐ ☐

Are you unhappy with what you have achieved in life? ☐ ☐

If you answered **Yes** to more than three questions it's time to learn
how to feel more positive about yourself.

Make a note of your score on your Real Life Diet on page 309; it
will be useful to compare it to your 'after' score, which you will complete in three months' time.

Now, take five minutes out, get a pen and find a comfortable place
to sit and relax. Now make a list of five things you like about yourself and another five you like about your body.

Five things I like about myself   **Five things I like about my body**

_____   _____

_____   _____

_____   _____

_____   _____

_____   _____

How to be positive

Being outgoing and optimistic is more likely to bring success than
spending time introspecting. There is plenty of evidence that those
who believe they will be successful usually are. So if you are short on
confidence make a point of indulging in some positive thinking for
ten minutes every morning when you wake up and before you go to
sleep at night. Get a vivid picture of your slim and attractive body

going through life being incredibly positive and see things through those positive eyes.

Spend time imagining yourself in ideal physical shape, looking and feeling great with good things happening to you. Maybe you are indulging in passionate encounters or enjoying the company of new friends. Perhaps your daydreams will centre round success in your studies or at work, or you want to look and feel attractive to others. Whatever you decide to focus on, make the images in your mind so realistic that you can actually feel you are the experiencing the situation. It may take some practice, but once you get the hang of it, it becomes like watching a movie. Remember, unless you feel positive about yourself you don't stand much chance of getting yourself into shape.

Pat yourself on the back

It also helps to keep a note of your daily achievements, however small. It is too easy to move on to the next thing, or even the next day, without acknowledging what you have actually accomplished. Again, we tend to fixate on the negative, our mistakes and things that perhaps we later regret. Making time to review your successes helps to build your self-confidence. Get yourself a notebook, and write in it on a daily basis as you would a diary. In the same way, as you begin to lose weight, keep a note of it each week and congratulate yourself.

Make yourself proud

Life can be so demanding that it's all too easy to go from day to day fulfilling your own needs without stopping to consider the needs of others. A big part of liking yourself is the reward that comes from helping to make other people's lives more pleasant. Why not team up with a friend and give them help and encouragement as they go through the Real Life Diet with you – you might be surprised how much of a buzz it will give you.

Living your dream

We don't always get what we dare to dream of without putting in a little effort. If you talk to six different people, you will probably find six quite different views on how to succeed in life and fulfil dreams. Some may even suggest that there is no point to dreaming, for fate will take charge of your destiny. We are each perfectly entitled to our own view, but there is now significant evidence to suggest that you can get much of what you wish for by applying specific techniques. Positive thinking and visualisation, when channelled correctly, can go a long way to getting you where you'd like to be, in the shape that you would like to be in. And there is scientific evidence to support this approach.

It is worth taking time out each day to visualise yourself just the way you would like to be. Experts believe we are at our most suggestive first thing in the morning when we wake and last thing at night just before going to sleep. So start and finish the day with a five- or ten-minute visualisation of yourself just the way you would like to be, slim, attractive, fit, successful, on a beach, with the partner of your dreams or whatever takes your fancy, and imagine living life as your ideal self. Visualising is an acquired skill, so if it doesn't happen in full Technicolor and your mind keeps wandering at first, stick at it, as you will eventually get the hang of it and hopefully start living your dreams. You have nothing to lose and it's a positive, fun and therapeutic way to begin and end the day. Regular visualisation of your ideal scene will help you lose weight, improve your fitness and love yourself a whole lot more.

CHAPTER 7

Are you stressed?

Do you ever pace around and find yourself eating more chocolate snacks or generally grazing as a comfort while distracted by your stresses? When stress becomes distressful we often lose our resolve to eat healthily, find it hard to love ourselves and that's when the rot sets in.

Up to a point, stress can actually be healthy, in that it keeps us alert and ready to face the day ahead. However, there is a fine line between stress and distress. Professor Hans Selye, the founder of modern research into stress, described it as 'the rate of wear and tear on the body'. He distinguished between good and bad stress. Good stress can be reasonably healthy as it stretches us to capacity and keeps us on our toes. However, when we reach the point of overload, the stress has an adverse effect leaving many of us feeling overwhelmed and under par.

We all have different ways of dealing with stress, and while some of us take it in our stride, others use methods of coping that can result in undesirable symptoms. Weight gain, as a result of comfort eating, or bingeing, is a classic side-effect of the 'too much on my plate syndrome', but it is not the only undesirable phenomenon. Other effects of stress can include depression, migraine headaches, panic attacks, fatigue, irritable bowel syndrome, a nervous rash or even recurrent thrush.

But the good news is you don't have to live like this. The important thing is to do regular stress checks to make sure you are keeping the balance between good and bad stress. If the scales are leaning towards the bad it's time to set in place a protective plan so your body is in the best possible state to stand up to stress and to take it in its stride. Take the stress test by answering Yes or No to the following questions:

How stressed are you?

	Yes	No
Are you tired all the time?	☐	☐
Do you have trouble sleeping or do you wake up in the middle of the night?	☐	☐
Do you crave sugary foods?	☐	☐
Do you keep bursting into tears?	☐	☐
Do you get frequent headaches?	☐	☐
Do you find it difficult to make up your mind?	☐	☐
Do you get butterflies in your stomach?	☐	☐
Do you feel anxious or on edge for no reason?	☐	☐
Do you feel overwhelmed?	☐	☐
Have you got emotional problems?	☐	☐
Are your family relationships strained?	☐	☐
Are you forgetful?	☐	☐
Is your digestive system upset?	☐	☐

	Yes	No
Is your appetite reduced?	☐	☐
Do you feel you have 'too much on your plate'?	☐	☐
Are you short-tempered?	☐	☐
Has your alcohol consumption increased?	☐	☐
Do you find it difficult to communicate with people?	☐	☐
Do you have little time for yourself?	☐	☐
Do you do fewer than three sessions of exercise per week?	☐	☐

If you answered **Yes** to more than 3 questions, the chances are you are suffering from stress overload. If you scored more than 6 **Yes** answers, you really need to take some urgent action to get back into the driving seat. First you need to look at any obvious triggers and deal with them as best you can. Then you can get started on my three-point protection plan to help you stand up to the pressure.

The three-point stress protection plan

1. Eat well

Stress is one of the most common causes of digestive upsets such as indigestion, bloating, IBS and heartburn. Some people eat less when they are stressed, but many more comfort eat and gradually gain weight as a result. Stress hormones can also dry up saliva, making swallowing difficult. A healthy, balanced diet will provide the necessary fuel you need to see you through the most difficult times. The Real Life Diet offers such a diet, but the following tips on eating well will also help reduce your stress levels.

- Consuming nutritious food little and often keeps blood sugar levels constant. Eat breakfast, lunch and dinner each day, with a wholesome mid-morning and mid-afternoon snack.

- Eat fresh, home-cooked foods wherever possible.

- Eat foods that are naturally sweet like dried fruit, fresh fruit, nuts and seeds, rather than foods with added sugar.

- Relax while you are eating and enjoy your food. Bolting food down or eating on the run can result in you swallowing too much air, which can lead to bloating.

- Cut down on tea and coffee. Try caffeine-free Rooibosch (Redbush) tea or coffee substitutes instead, or herbal teas.

2. Get moving

All too often our exercise regimes go out of the window at the first sign of stress. This is the opposite of what we should be doing, as physical exercise is one of the best stress busters there is. Research shows that regular activity helps to speed up the metabolism and encourages the release of endorphins, the body's own feel-good hormones, which improve our mood and put us in a better frame of mind for dealing with difficult situations.

- 30 minutes of exercise most days of the week is a healthy goal to aim for.

- Choose an activity you like, as you are more likely to stick to it. Walking, cycling, jogging, dancing and swimming are all good choices.

- If you prefer exercising with other people, you could join an exercise class, work out to an exercise video or simply get singing and dancing to your favourite music.

- It will really help to note down how much you do so you can take pride in your achievements.

3. Sleep well

While you are asleep your body gets down to the essential processes of cell repair and rejuvenation, so a good night's sleep is essential if you are to wake up ready to face the day ahead. If you can't get to sleep or feel sleepy all the time, chances are you're suffering from stress overload. Waking up in the middle of the night and fitful dreams are other common signs.

- Try to get at least eight hours' sleep a night (you will know if you function well on less than this) and if your sleep is disturbed because of the stress take some valerian, a natural herb that will help you to relax.

- Establish a regular sleep pattern by going to bed and getting up at the same time every day.

- Avoid eating and exercising too close to bedtime.

- Taking a short power nap after lunch can help to recharge your batteries.

Real life story

Photographer, **Danniel**, 55, from Sydney had battled with his weight, stress and a number of health issues for many years.

❝ I had a busy, challenging work life. I had yo-yo dieted for 20 years but all I had to show for it was failure, high cholesterol and gout. I constantly felt annoyed and frustrated. Maryon read me the riot act many times and I resisted. But one day I woke up and said to myself "enough is enough". I decided to cut out all the junk and switch to the healthy food Maryon had suggested. I began walking every day for an hour, and gradually built up the intensity of the exercise and the weight began to fall off. I also reorganised my business and eventually took up t'ai chi, which began to balance my life mentally.

➤

I lost 44 lb (20 kg) in six months. I began to feel like my old self and so much younger. My self-esteem returned and I bought a new wardrobe of clothes. My blood tests now show normal levels on all aspects – in fact I have since been taken off my cholesterol tablets by my doctor and haven't had any gout since the new regime. I still love my food and go out to eat often, but certain food categories have been reduced or excluded. I continue to exercise regularly, and enjoy what has become my new, balanced way of life. I thoroughly enjoy my work now and I even teach t'ai chi. It's a complete turnaround. **"**

Make time for yourself to beat stress

Making time for yourself is not just a nice idea, it is essential, especially if your life is busy and full. The ability to 'switch off' and refresh is the key to well-being, but it is not always as easy as it sounds. If you are preoccupied, wound up and tense, it can be hard to see the benefits of taking time out. Being able to relax thoroughly is actually an acquired skill – which for some of us takes a little practice – but all that is required is some time (around 15 to 20 minutes a day), and a comfortable space in which to spend that time. Relaxation is becoming more important as many of us continue to live life in the fast lane. The Pzizz machine is a little portable unit that provides tailor made relaxation programmes whenever it suits you, and is a great discovery, that I have to admit I now carry around with me at all times. It provides several different proven techniques to give you the most refreshing and revitalising 'nap' possible. It is a blend of NLP with especially composed music, sound effects and a binaural beat to induce a wonderfully relaxed stage. The new guided meditation CD produced by Sue Fisher Hendry also comes highly recommended and is available by mail order (see page 84 for details). Once you have learned the art of relaxation you can practise it at any time, and, best of all, it is free. To get started try the simple exercise in the box below or you might like to try a more formal method of relaxation, such as yoga or meditation. If you are not used to switching off, try using the excellent collection of guided *Mediations and Creative Visualisation* by Sue Fisher Hendry. This is available from the mail order service on 020 7631 4235 or from the shop at www.naturalhealth.com.

Yoga and meditation are both popular techniques, which allow you to practise mind over matter. Massage is a useful tool and many of the martial arts like t'ai chi are therapeutic too. You will find further information in the Recommended Reading and Further Information and Useful Addresses and Websites sections on pages 321 and 323.

Let it go

You will need to find a quiet space where you can confidently switch off. If necessary, put the answerphone on, or take the phone off the hook. Let people know that you don't want to be disturbed for a while, and put on some comfortable, loose clothes. Either lie down on a mat, a soft carpet or firm bed. Make sure that you are comfortable with the room temperature and lighting. You can play some calming music in the background. Once you feel comfortable, do the following, step by step:

- Place a pillow under your head, and stretch out full length. Relax your arms and your lower jaw.

- Take a few slow, deep breaths before you begin.

- Then concentrate on relaxing your muscles, starting with the toes on one foot and then the other. Gradually work your way slowly up your body, going through all the muscle groups.

➤

- As you do so, first tense each group of muscles and then relax them, taking care to breathe deeply as you relax.

- When you reach your head, and your face feels relaxed, remain in the relaxed position for 10 to 15 minutes, perhaps imagining yourself walking along a beautiful beach or one of your favourite places.

- Gradually allow yourself to 'come to'. Roll over on to your side, sit up gradually and slowly drink a glass of water while you allow yourself to fully return to real life.

Top stress busters

Here are some tips to help keep stress at bay and your mood buoyant:

- Make sure you have some sacred time for yourself for meditation and relaxation.

- Tell your family how you feel and ask for their support.

- If your stress comes from work, discuss with colleagues how you can make changes, or if you are self-employed you will need to re-evaluate.

- Try to get away; even it's only for a few days.

- Learn not to take on too much.

- Prioritise your responsibilities and see if you can offload or delegate some of the less important tasks.

- Eat regular, wholesome meals and have a supply of nutritious snacks at the ready.

- Make sure you are getting enough magnesium. Good sources include fruit and dark green leafy vegetables.

- Avoid caffeine in the form of tea, coffee, chocolate and cola as it acts as a stimulant.

- Keep your alcohol consumption to a minimum as it can also act as a stimulant and disturb your sleep.

- Ask your partner or close friend to give you a massage.

- Watch an entertaining film or read a good book.

- Make sure you find things to laugh about.

- Make a point of singing in the bath!

Real life story

Michelle Grant had sorted out her PMS with my help ten years ago, but she became perimenopausal in her early forties and her life became stressful. She came back for help as she felt she had lost control.

❦ I had been coasting along nicely since sorting out my severe PMS in the early 1990s. I wasn't really paying much attention to myself as I was too busy dealing with my family. My teenage daughter was going through a wild child phase and my husband was working shifts and was stressed. I was in a daze one day when I got knocked off my bicycle by a car and it was only then that I realised how badly things had slipped. My mood swings and depression had returned and I was feeling incredibly tired.

I got back in touch with Maryon who suggested I follow the Real Life Diet, including a new supplement regime. She insisted I start exercising again and practising relaxation techniques, plus have regular massage and generally making time for myself.

➤

I am far less stressed and can now support my family with a new-found energy. I changed my career, which was rewarding in itself, and am now in the process of retraining, which I could never have done before. Best of all I feel back in control and that my life is in a much better balance. **'**

CHAPTER 8

De-clutter your life

Feeling overwhelmed by clutter in your life is often the perfect excuse for a bout of comfort eating. Sorting out clutter at home and at work has an unburdening and energising effect that helps to promote the weight loss process.

Whether you are out at work all day or at home looking after the kids there always seems to be too much to do and before you know it backlogs accumulate. Your life has become cluttered with seemingly important tasks, obligations to friends and families, and maybe an untidy home and work place. Start to deal with this weighty problem now by answering Yes or No to the questions below to assess just how much clutter there is in your life:

Check out your clutter

	Yes	**No**
Do you have piles of paper in random places around the house?	☐	☐
Do you have to have a major tidy-up before you welcome guests into your home?	☐	☐

Yes No

Are you a hoarder? ☐ ☐

Do you find it difficult to part with old possessions even if they are worn out because of sentimental value? ☐ ☐

Do you always put tidying up off for another day? ☐ ☐

Are your handbags/briefcases stuffed full of random papers and objects? ☐ ☐

Are your cupboards and drawers untidy? ☐ ☐

Do you stuff things into cupboards to get them out of the way? ☐ ☐

Do you keep old newspapers and magazines? ☐ ☐

Is your desk at work piled high with papers? ☐ ☐

Do you feel that you are constantly chasing your tail to keep on top of things? ☐ ☐

Are you seeing less of your friends than you used to? ☐ ☐

Are you aware that your clutter affects your mood? ☐ ☐

If you answered **Yes** to more than 3 questions it's probably time for some physical and possibly mental spring cleaning. Don't forget to put your score on your Real Life Diet on page 309.

Clear out your home

There's nothing more draining and depressing than an untidy living space. According to Chinese wisdom, clutter represents blocked energy and can quickly lower your spirits. Choose a room that you spend a lot of time in and start clearing it out. Look around and if something doesn't help lift your mood or you have not used it in the past 12 months be ruthless. Get rid of it and create some empty space.

If you find it really hard to do this, try asking yourself what is the worst thing that could happen if you get rid of it. If all else fails employ the services of a Clutter Doctor to get you started (see Useful Addresses and Websites on page 323).

Once the throwing out is done, the next step is to get cleaning. Move all the furniture, vacuum behind it and dust every surface. Aim to make the room as welcoming and relaxing as you can. Go on to clear every room in the same way.

Finally, treat yourself to some new house-plants. Some, such as spider plants, gerbera and peace lilies, can help to absorb pollutants from cleaning products, paints and synthetic fibres.

Review your friendships

According to the life coach experts it's not people that are toxic but relationships and those with your friends or family may need reviewing from time to time. Healthy relationships thrive on good communication and mutual understanding while bad ones fester with resentment and unspoken feelings. If you don't love your relationships, it is hard to love yourself and this usually has a major impact on your physical appearance and your weight.

If, for example, you are surrounded by friends who take but never seem to give anything back, it's time for you to ask yourself why you are allowing this to happen. You may like rescuing people but if they don't contribute to the relationship you might decide to stop being a rescuer. You should also aim to set boundaries and decide what you are and are not willing to accept within your relationships.

When it comes to loved ones and partners if things get difficult try to concentrate on their good points and what brought you together in the first place, rather than what is driving you mad at the moment. Try to support them emotionally through the bad times as well as the good. Remember also that very few relationships thrive on constant togetherness, so try to respect each other's need for space and time alone.

De-clutter your work space

A healthy desk equals a healthy mind so get rid of the clutter and watch your energy levels rise. Keep only work in progress on your desk. It will help focus your mind. Look at each piece of paper as it arrives. Deal with it, file it or bin it. Take stretch breaks every hour. Take a walk round the office and you will return to your desk revived and more able to concentrate. Essential oils can also help to clear your mind to enhance your working day. If you start to feel the pressure put a couple of drops of the following oils on a tissue and breathe in deeply. Try orange, if you're feeling down; lavender, if you're dreading the next few hours; camomile, if you are a workaholic or a perfectionist; bergamot, if you're suffering from a sense of humour failure; and melissa, if panic strikes.

A de-cluttered work space will help you to concentrate your energies on the Real Life Diet and achieve success.

De-clutter your mind

A cluttered mind can stifle creative thought, deplete energy levels and lower your spirits, making it hard to love yourself. The secret is to try and empty your mind from time to time to give yourself the chance to recharge your batteries, which will reinvigorate and rejuvenate body and soul.

If you are starting to feel guilty about taking restorative time out just for you, don't. This is not an indulgence but rather a practical way of ensuring you keep a healthy balance in your life. Relaxation can be difficult to achieve. Most of us are so used to being tense and wound up that we find letting go almost impossible. For a simple way to relax every day, wherever you are, follow the exercise described in the box below.

Breathe deeply to increase your energy levels

It's simple, it's free and it's amazingly effective. Learning to breathe deeply via alternate nostril breathing the way the yogis do maximises oxygen intake and can really rev up energy levels. It floods the body with rich oxygenated air, gets rid of stale carbon dioxide, sharpens the mind and wakes you up like nothing else.

- Find a quiet place and sit down comfortably.

- Extend the index finger and thumb of your right hand.

- Rest your thumb against your right nostril and breathe in through your left nostril for a count of four.

- Close both nostrils for a count of four.

- Open your right nostril and exhale deeply for a count of four.

- Repeat exercise eight times, starting with the other nostril each time.

CHAPTER 9

Boosting your libido

Having good sex regularly is regarded as an essential part of a well-balanced life for many people. It keeps us feeling happy, loved and in good physical shape. As an added bonus, an hour of active lovemaking uses up at least 150 calories and helps to keep many groups of muscles toned and in good shape.

When it comes to levels of libido there is no such thing as normal. It varies from person to person and what seems low to you may be perfectly acceptable to someone else. Also, it is not uncommon to lose interest in sex as the years go by. Until now you may have thought that this is part of the ageing process and have to put up with it, but happily this is not the case.

Low levels of important nutrients, particularly mixed vitamin B and magnesium, which is more common than you might imagine, childbirth, sleepless nights, the daily stresses and strains of work and life all take their toll and you may not feel much like having sex. Thyroid problems, diabetes, weight gain and hormonal changes at times of the menstrual cycle or the menopause can also affect your love life. But the good news is there is plenty you can do to rekindle your desire. The first thing to do is to listen to your body to see what could be at the root of your waning libido by taking the test below, and then decide on the best course of action.

How's your libido?

Take the test, marking yes or no in the relevant column:

	Yes	No
Have you lost your sex drive?	☐	☐
Do you have sex as often as you used to?	☐	☐
Do you make excuses in order to avoid having sex?	☐	☐
Do you fake orgasms?	☐	☐
Have you stopped looking forward to having sex?	☐	☐
Has your enjoyment of sex diminished?	☐	☐
Do you prefer chocolate to sex?	☐	☐
Are you too tired for sex?	☐	☐
Are you too busy dealing with the children to have sex?	☐	☐
Do you feel less sexy?	☐	☐
Has your physical shape changed?	☐	☐
Have you stopped being your partner's lover?	☐	☐
Do you find sex painful?	☐	☐
Have you stopped communicating to your partner on an intimate level?	☐	☐
Do you no longer fancy your partner?	☐	☐
(if female) Is your vagina dry?	☐	☐
(if male) Do you have trouble sustaining an erection?	☐	☐
Would you rather watch football than have sex?	☐	☐

If you answered yes to more than 3 of the questions, try the following to help give your sex life a boost. Then turn to page 309 to enter your score on your Real Life Diet.

How to boost your sex life

Watch your weight: Apart from being unhealthy, carrying excess pounds is bad for self-esteem, which will do nothing for your sex life. Losing weight can also help improve hormone function especially in women. So one of the wonderful side-effects of successfully following the Real Life Diet could be a hugely improved love life!

Sexy foods: Oysters and other seafood are well known for their aphrodisiac qualities, and chocolate is believed to stimulate the production of endorphins, the body's own feel-good hormones. Celery and parsnips may not spring to mind as sexy vegetables but both are good sources of androdestenol, a substance believed to mimic human pheromones – our own built-in sexual fragrance designed to attract mates.

Watch the alcohol: A glass of wine or champagne can be one of the greatest aphrodisiacs but take care you don't overdo it. It may increase your desire but could end up reducing your performance.

Move it: The fitter you are the higher your sex drive is likely to be, so get moving. Exercise also encourages the production of endorphins. Dancing with your partner, using plenty of body and eye contact, can be especially stimulating. Keep moving for at least 20 minutes to allow time for the feel-good hormones to kick in.

Get in touch: One of the simplest yet most effective sex boosters lies within easy reach – at your fingertips. Treat each other to a sensual massage. Turn on the music, dim the lights and start to gently touch each other. Intuitive touching, stroking and kneading are all that's needed but using essential oils, such as jasmine, rose, clary sage, sandalwood, neroli, ylang ylang and frankincense, may heighten the experience.

Talk to each other: Taking your partner for granted is an easy habit to slip into, but it's also guaranteed to create a distance between you. Try to spend some time together, perhaps on a special weekend away, and talk about what is important to you both. This should bring you emotionally closer, which in turn will bring you sexually closer as well.

Say it with flowers: If your relationship is less than healthy, a dose of Bach Flower Remedies may bring back the loving spark. Wild Rose remedy is believed to renew interest in life and boost vitality, while Olive is thought to have revitalising properties. Larch is the one to go for if you've lost confidence in your ability to make love.

Supplement it: As you might be able to guess from the name, horny goat weed has a reputation as a natural aphrodisiac. It has a testosterone-like effect in that it stimulates desire and sexual activity in women, as well as increasing sperm production and increased sensitivity in the sensory nerves of the penis in men. Research has shown that a 600-mg dose of horny goat weed can inhibit an enzyme called acetylcholinesterase (AChE), which stops neurotransmission needed for speedy responses in the neuromuscular system. By inhibiting AChE, horny goat weed is able to support higher levels of neurotransmitters associated with sexual arousal.

ArginMax is another specially formulated natural supplement and is available in both male and female formulations (see page 128 for details). Five different double-blind placebo controlled studies, conducted at respected institutions throughout the world, have credited ArginMax with an 80 per cent and 75 per cent improvement in men's and women's libido respectively. ArginMax for Women is a combination of L-Arginine, ginseng, ginkgo, and 14 essential vitamins and minerals that work together to support sexual function and enjoyment. In addition, it provides a daily multivitamin that includes important antioxidants and the minerals calcium, iron and zinc.

ArginMax for Men is a premium performance formula of L-Arginine, ginseng, ginkgo, antioxidant vitamins A, C and E, and vitamin B complex that helps to support sexual fitness, and provide men with their recommended daily amount of 13 vitamins and minerals such as selenium, zinc and niacin.

It may take at least a month to notice any difference at all, but within three or four months you should both notice a dramatic improvement in your libido.

St John's wort has also been shown to help boost libido.

Ginkgo biloba boosts circulation to the extremities and could therefore help to get your partner in the mood.

Muira puama is a Brazilian herb, also known as potency wood, which has long been used as an aphrodisiac by tribespeople in the Amazon.

Damiana has been used as a natural aphrodisiac for thousands of years in Latin American countries. It is said to increase sensitivity of nerve endings in the genitals and to help reduce anxiety and depression when these are linked with sexual difficulties.

Real life story

Ruth Harvey was 36 when she first came to see me. She owned a hairdressing salon and had two young children. She was experiencing unpleasant symptoms following a hysterectomy and had put on a lot of weight.

❝ I was given a radical hysterectomy in my mid-30s, which left me feeling like I had lost control of my body, and gained a lot of weight, which made me feel awful. I visited my GP, who was not very sympathetic and prescribed HRT, which helped my night sweats but made other symptoms worse and made it impossible to shift the weight.

I got into a terrible state emotionally and became desperate as no one really seemed to understand what I was going through. Then I saw an article about the NHAS and arranged to see Maryon. She suggested I made some dietary changes to help me lose weight and balance my hormones. The results were almost immediate and I started to feel better.

I have now been following the Real Life Diet for about 18 months. I no longer use any HRT and am back to my old self. I've been told that I look great and I certainly feel good. I've lost weight, got myself back into shape, my cravings for sweets are gone and I feel like my life is balanced again. Best of all, my libido, which was non-existent, has returned, and my husband keeps telling me how delighted he is to have his wife back. ❞

CHAPTER · **10**

Eat to beat... common conditions sorted

Many of us walk around suffering with a whole host of common health problems, without realising for a minute that there may be very workable and natural solutions out there. Often debilitating symptoms, which affect everything from our energy levels through to personal relationships and self-esteem, are just a result of us not getting the balance right in our diet and lifestyle, and they can get progressively worse unless we take positive action. Being distracted by symptoms often results in us caring less about our appearance, and pain and discomfort can affect our desire or ability to exercise, which makes problems with overweight harder to deal with. It's hard to concentrate on a sensible eating and exercise plan when you are dealing with the often overwhelming problems caused by your particular condition.

More than 20 years of sitting in the hot seat at the Natural Health Advisory Service (NHAS) has taught me that most of these symptoms can be overcome naturally within a matter of months with the right self-help measures. This section is designed to give you some basic advice to get you on the road to recovery and ready to tackle the Real Life Diet as described in Part Two of this book. As well as promoting weight loss, the Real Life Diet will continue to help you address and resolve common conditions, leaving you feeling good as well as looking good.

You may wish to only read the sections of this chapter that apply to you, so here is a mini contents list to help you navigate your way around:

Irritable bowel syndrome (IBS)

IBS or irritable bowel syndrome affects an estimated 20 per cent of people in the UK and it can make life a misery. Typical symptoms include constipation or diarrhoea, or a combination of the two, abdominal pain, bloating, excessive wind, mucus or slime in the stool, nausea or loss of appetite and indigestion.

CAUSES: Stress, a bad diet, severe gastroenteritis and prolonged use of antibiotics are thought to be factors but symptoms often occur with no one determining factor. It is thought that in most cases a combination of triggers as well as genetic factors could be at play.

Help yourself

- Follow an exclusion diet, which means avoiding common allergenic foods such as wheat, dairy, eggs and citrus fruits, for a set period of time and then introducing them one by one to help pinpoint the likely culprit. All the advice you need on how to proceed is found in Part Two of this book, which deals in detail with how to exclude and reintroduce foods into your diet.

- Take a probiotic supplement to help balance the good and bad bacteria in your gut, which will help relieve wind.

- If you are constipated add two tablespoons of organic golden linseeds to your morning cereal. Magnesium amino acid chelate supplements can also help improve bowel function.

- If you suffer with diarrhoea take a strong B complex tablet daily.

- Aloe vera gel or liquid can help to keep the digestive tract healthy.

- Digestive enzymes can help in the short term.

- Charcoal tablets can offer immediate relief from bloating but should not be taken on a daily basis or at the same time as nutritional supplements, as they can inhibit the absorption of nutrients.

- Peppermint oil capsules can also help ease intestinal spasms and bloating.

Further advice is available in the book *No More IBS* (see page 322).

Thrush

Thrush is an infection caused by candida albicans, a yeast that lives in places such as the vagina and anus. It thrives in warm moist areas so can also occur in the groin or mouth. Symptoms in women include a thick white vaginal discharge, a vaginal itch, a burning sensation while passing urine and sometimes a rash. Men can also get thrush and symptoms include redness and itching at the tip of the penis and under the foreskin.

CAUSES: Thrush is usually caused by a disturbance in the balance between the good and bad bacteria in the gut. Being run down or taking antibiotics can lower your defences while menstrual changes, pregnancy, the menopause or taking the Pill can also trigger symptoms.

Help yourself

- Avoid products that contain yeast, such as bread. Foods such as blue cheese, mushrooms, dried fruits, and fermented drinks such as wine and beer can also encourage fungal growth.

- Steer clear of acidic foods, such as citrus fruits, and spicy foods, as acid can destroy the alkalinity of your gut, creating a breeding ground for fungi.

- Candida thrives on sugar too, so give sugary foods a miss.

- Replenish your stores of good bacteria by eating live yogurt and flush out your system by drinking at least 2 litres (3½ pints) of water every day.

- Boosting the immune system by supplementing your diet with zinc and vitamin C. The herb echinacea may also help keep candida at bay.

- Always wipe from front to back after going to the loo and wear cotton underwear.

- Avoid wearing tight jeans.

Cystitis

Cystitis is an inflammation of the bladder wall and is usually the result of a bacterial infection. Typical symptoms include a frequent need to go to the loo often accompanied by a painful stinging sensation. You may experience lower abdominal pain and, in more serious cases, weakness and fever. Your urine may also be cloudy and strong smelling.

CAUSES: In around 50 per cent of cases the organism E coli is the culprit. It normally lives in the bowel but vigorous sex or wiping from back to front after going to the loo can mean it penetrates the urethra and works its way into the bladder. Tight clothing, which puts pressure on the urethra, is another factor, while vaginal deodorants and disinfectants can also bring on symptoms.

Help yourself

- Drink plenty of liquids, especially water, throughout the day. Try to drink the equivalent of a glass of water every hour while symptoms are acute to flush your system through.

- Drink unsweetened cranberry juice or cranberry extract. It contains hippuric acid, which actually inhibits the bacteria responsible for cystitis from adhering to the lining of the bladder and urinary tract.

- Dissolving a teaspoon of bicarbonate soda in a glass of water and then drinking it can help to make your urine less acidic.

- After sex or a bowel movement wash yourself carefully with warm, unperfumed soapy water, wiping yourself from front to back to wash away any lurking germs.

- Pass urine when you need to, making sure you completely empty your bladder. Always go as soon as you can after sex.

- Use a natural lubricant during sex to reduce friction and bruising.

Premenstrual syndrome (PMS)

Premenstrual syndrome or PMS is a collection of symptoms that occur from around two weeks before your period, which tail off as bleeding begins. Symptoms include anxiety, irritability, mood swings, tension, depression, tearfulness, loss of libido and forgetfulness. Breast tenderness, headaches, a craving for sweet things, bloating and fatigue are the most common physical symptoms.

CAUSES: The experts remain divided on the causes. Some put it down to a hormonal imbalance while others maintain it has more to do with fluctuations in brain chemicals or even that it could all be in the mind. In my experience at the NHAS, however, I find that while these imbalances may be factors there are other things at play such as nutritional and lifestyle deficiencies. Once these are corrected sufferers experience a relief in symptoms in a matter of months.

Help yourself

- Eat little and often to maintain optimum blood-sugar levels, and to keep a good supply of nutrients flowing to the brain and nervous system.

- Make sure you eat your daily five portions of fruit and veg, and two portions of oily fish a week. Good choices include mackerel, herring, salmon, pilchards and sardines.

- Eat some protein, such as chicken, fish, lean meat, low-fat cheese, eggs or a vegetarian protein, with your lunch and dinner.

- Drink herbal teas rather than tea, coffee and cola or other drinks containing caffeine.

- Avoid sodium, salt and salty food – salt tends to drag fluid into cells, which can make you feel bloated. Use fresh herbs, garlic, ginger and black pepper for flavouring.

- Replace sugary biscuits and cakes with naturally sweet foods such as dried or fresh fruit, nuts and seeds.

- Cut back your intake of dairy foods to the equivalent of milk on your cereal, milk in your drinks plus one other serving of dairy a day, such as yoghurt or cheese.

- The herbal supplement agnus castus and a good multivitamin and mineral supplement (such as Optivite, page 126) can help regulate the menstrual cycle and balance hormone levels.

- Aim for three or four aerobic exercise sessions a week. Cycling, swimming, brisk walking, jogging, skipping or a gym workout are all good choices.

Further solutions are available in the book *No More PMS* (see page 322).

Real life story

Janet Slater was 39 when she first came to see me. She had gained 22 lb (10 kg), which she was finding difficult to shift, as well as suffering with PMS and a very short menstrual cycle. She had a demanding career as a finance director and was prevented from finding a partner because she felt so out of sorts.

❛ I was on the verge of going to hospital each time my period arrived because of the severe pain and clotting. And they would come so often. I felt incredibly sick for two days and then the pain and the bleeding began. My breasts were sore, I was irritable, depressed, anxious and spent a good deal of time comfort eating, which was probably why I had gained

➤

so much weight. Maryon got to work giving me a detailed diet, supplement and exercise programme to follow, based on the Real Life Diet. I was amazed that within the first month the breast pain was gone completely. Within three months I had my first pain-free period ever, I ran a half marathon, which I had only ever thought I could do in my dreams and I had lost nearly a stone (7 kg) without dieting. I took some time off work to decide what I wanted to do in the long term now that I was feeling so much better and having completely regular periods. Maryon got me doing some visualising and I have met a wonderful man, so now have a very happy relationship. I'm back to my normal weight and in better shape than ever. My life is so different now, worlds apart from how it was before and I really feel like I have the balance right. 〞

Menopause

Menopause literally means your last menstrual period and the average age at which a woman reaches menopause is 51. In the years leading up to this event, your body goes through a series of changes, which are known as the perimenopause, meaning around the time and before the onset of the menopause. Symptoms include hot flushes, night sweats, headaches, urinary infections and genital irritation. Mood swings, forgetfulness, anxiety and lack of concentration are also common. Until recently many doctors were prescribing hormone replacement therapy (HRT) for long-term use, but in the light of international research findings HRT is now tending to being prescribed only for short-term use. At the NHAS we have pioneered an effective scientifically proven non-drug approach to the menopause, which also helps to protect the heart, the bones and memory in the longer term.

CAUSES: As you enter your forties your ovaries start to slow down, egg production gradually stops and oestrogen, the hormone produced by the ovaries during your child-bearing years, also starts to drop. As oestrogen levels drop still further, usually in the early fifties, many women start to experience the aforementioned symptoms, which can last for months or linger for years.

Help yourself

- Eat plenty of fresh fruit and veg, dairy products, and eight glasses of water a day. A glass of cold water at the beginning of a hot flush will help to return the body's thermostat back to normal.

- Try to avoid sugar and junk foods, which can block the uptake of vital nutrients.

- A diet rich in phytoestrogens (substances similar to human oestrogen which occur naturally in plants) can help relieve symptoms, as well as helping to protect against heart disease and osteoporosis. The richest sources are soya products, especially soya milk, tofu and soya flour. Other sources include organic linseeds, lentils, chickpeas, mung beans, sunflower, pumpkin and sesame seeds, and green and yellow vegetables. You should aim to eat around 100 mg of phytoestrogens a day.

- To relieve hot flushes wear several layers of thin clothing, which you can peel off if you start to feel hot. Use lightweight bedclothes, which you can arrange according to the temperature and go for cotton nightwear. Hot drinks, alcohol and spicy foods, which can aggravate flushing, should also be avoided.

- Try to spend 15–20 minutes relaxing each day to keep stress levels down and hot flushes at bay. Research shows these simple measures will reduce hot flushes by as much as 60 per cent.

- Aim to exercise for at least half an hour five times a week. You need to do weight-bearing exercise that is also aerobic. Good choices include brisk walking, jogging, racket sports, dancing, aerobics and skipping.

- Take daily supplements of the multivitamin and mineral supplement Gynovite and Novogen red clover (see pages 126 and 127) or Arkopharma Phyto Soya (see page 129) as these have been shown to help normalise hormone levels and reduce the flushing.

- If you suffer with a dry vagina use Pharma Nords Omega 7 daily and Phyto Soya vaginal gel twice a week.

Further solutions can be found in the book *Beat Menopause Naturally*, which is part of the new Natural Menopause Kit. This can be ordered from www.askmaryonstewart.com or www.naturalmenopause.com.

Prostate problems

From mid-life onwards most men can expect some degree of prostate enlargement (a swelling of the small gland that lies beneath the bladder). As the prostate gland enlarges it compresses the urethra – the outlet tube that passes through and also pushes up on the base of the bladder. This produces symptoms such as outflow obstruction, poor flow, dribbling, incomplete emptying and other symptoms of frequency, urgency sometimes with incontinence and a need to pass water at night (nocturia).

The condition is usually benign but occasionally urinary problems can be the first sign of prostate cancer, especially if there is also blood in the urine, so you should always check out symptoms with your GP.

CAUSES: It is part of the natural ageing process but can be controlled with adequate knowledge.

Help yourself

- Try following a low fat diet with at least five servings of fruit and veg a day. Zinc-rich foods such as seafood, whole grains, bran, pumpkin seeds, garlic and pulses may also help.

- Limit your fluid intake if you are drinking excessively, especially tea, coffee and alcohol, all of which have diuretic effects.

- Increase your intake of nuts and seeds, particularly pumpkin seeds; both contain essential fatty acids needed to make prostaglandins, substances vital for prostate health.

- You could also try supplementing your diet with the herbal remedy saw palmetto, which helps to control the bladder, and Trinovin, which has been shown to reduce prostate problems (see page 128). Extract of rye grass has also been used with some success in the treatment of prostate-related disorders.

Osteoporosis prevention

Sometimes known as brittle bone disease, osteoporosis happens when calcium, the mineral in bones, and collagen, the gluey protein that helps strengthen them, are lost. As a result the fine honeycomb texture of healthy bone becomes full of gaping holes. Osteoporosis is often dubbed the 'silent disease' with many women being unaware they have osteoporosis until they trip up over a pavement or stumble against a kitchen cupboard and end up with a broken hip or wrist.

CAUSES: Healthy bones are built in childhood and are at their most dense in our twenties. From around our mid thirties we start to lose bone at about one per cent a year for both women and men as part of the natural ageing process. In women this loss of bone speeds up to two or three per cent around the years of the menopause. This happens because of the natural drop in oestrogen, a hormone essential for bone health, at this time of life. This is one of the main reasons why middle-aged women are more vulnerable to osteoporosis than men. The weakened bones lose their ability to absorb shock and eventually become so fragile that even a small knock or fall can cause a fracture.

Help yourself

- Watch your diet. The two most important minerals for bone health are calcium (found in sardines, dairy foods, nuts, seeds, beans and green leafy vegetables) and magnesium (found in whole foods, nuts and seafood).

- Consider taking a 500 mg calcium supplement. Teenagers and woman under the age of 45 need an intake of at least 1,000 mg of calcium per day, and it is not always easy to be sure you are getting it through your diet. Taking supplements can be useful for older members of your family as well as those who are housebound or who feel they are not getting enough calcium from their diet.

- Vitamin D (found in egg yolk and oily fish) helps the body absorb calcium – and as vitamin D is produced in the body through the action of sunlight on the skin, sunshine is also important. About 20–30 minutes' exposure of the face and arms a day in the summer months should provide you with enough vitamin D for the health of your bones.

- Be careful not to have too much animal protein, salt or caffeine, as in excessive quantities these can reduce your body's ability to absorb or retain calcium.

- Smoking should be avoided as it can have a toxic effect on bone and may lead to an early menopause in women.

- You should also watch what you drink although the good news is that a moderate intake of one to two glasses of wine a day may have beneficial effects on the skeleton as well as the heart.

- Over the past ten years there has been a huge amount of interest in plant phytoestrogens. In humans they act like weaker forms of oestrogen, so may help protect against bone loss by mimicking to a much lesser degree, the effects of this hormone. Good sources include soya beans, soya products such as tofu and soya milk, and to a lesser degree lentils, chickpeas, mung beans and golden linseed.

- According to the experts exercise plays a vital part in building strong bones when we are younger and helping to maintain bone density, as we grow older. High impact or weight-bearing exercise, which puts pressure on the bones, is the most beneficial. Running, jogging, brisk walking, lifting weights in the gym, skipping and racquet sports are all good choices. Try to exercise at least three times a week for a minimum of 20 minutes.

Migraine

Migraine is usually classified into two different types – common migraine and classical migraine. With common migraine there is little or no warning of an attack. The pain develops slowly into a throbbing ache, which can be aggravated by movement or noise. Classical migraines are usually preceded by what is known as an aura – a collection of warning symptoms, which develop before an attack and can last for 10–60 minutes. These include visual disturbances, such as flashing lights or zigzag patterns, general blurring and even partial loss of sight. Both types are often accompanied by nausea and vomiting.

CAUSES: A migraine attack is thought to be the result of changes in neurotransmitters and blood vessels in the brain, but what exactly causes these changes is still open to debate. There are certain known triggers such as stress, foods such as cheese, alcohol and chocolate, lack of food or irregular meals, fatigue and hormonal factors such as periods and the menopause. Menstrual migraines are thought to be related to the drop in oestrogen at this time of the month.

Help yourself

- Avoid stress and do some sort of formal relaxation every day. Yoga and meditation are good choices. If you feel stress starting to get the better of you go for a walk or do some deep breathing.

- Never skip meals. Try to eat wholesome foods little and often to maintain blood sugar levels.

- Try to identify your triggers by cutting out the foods associated with migraine from your diet and seeing what makes a difference.

- Keep a migraine diary to see if there is any recurring pattern to your attacks. Use the Migrastick, the Arkopharma product, made from 100% natural essential oils of mint and lavender, that has been shown in clinical studies to reduce the pain caused the headaches and migraine.

- If you smoke, give it up.

- Taking an essential fatty acid supplement can help by reducing red blood cell clumping, which is associated with headaches.

- Take regular aerobic exercise – at least 30 minutes most days of the week.

- Chewing some ginger, either root or crystallised, can help to bring relief.

- The herb feverfew has been shown to help.

- Avoid getting dehydrated by drinking at least eight glasses of water a day.

- Complementary therapies such as massage, acupuncture and reflexology may help to keep attacks at bay.

Heart disease

Whether it is hardening of the arteries, high blood pressure or elevated cholesterol levels, the chances are that millions of us will be affected by heart disease in some way as we age, unless we work to prevent it. The elevation of blood pressure puts us at increased risk of having a stroke. The mechanisms behind these diseases are damage to the walls of the arteries that are subjected to the increase in pressure. The artery wall becomes thickened, the lining damaged and more prone to cholesterol deposits, particularly if the blood cholesterol level is raised. There is a strong association with the type of fat in the diet and high cholesterol. About one-third of the cholesterol in the blood is derived from the cholesterol we eat. The remainder is made in the liver and the amount made is determined by both genetic and dietary factors.

CAUSES: There are many minor causes of high blood pressure, including genetic factors as well as factors related to our diet, environment and general health. Being overweight, hormonal changes and the tendency to retain sodium salt are all factors that contribute to raised blood pressure. High intakes of saturated animal fats add to our risk of heart disease, probably because of the increased production of bad cholesterol by the liver, and may cause other blood changes, encouraging the deposit of that cholesterol on to the walls of our arteries. It is also recognised that increased levels of homocysteine, which occurs when there is a deficiency of folic acid and to a lesser degree vitamins B6 and B12, is responsible for blocking the arteries, which subsequently leads to heart attack and stroke.

Help yourself

- Have a daily serving of soya milk and a product such as Flora Pro Activ yogurt, which have both been shown to help lower cholesterol levels.

- Steer clear of salty foods and don't add salt to your food at the table or to your cooking.

- Sprinkle organic linseeds over your breakfast cereals.

- Keep your weight down.

- Don't smoke – it could mean the difference between life and death.

- Cut your intake of animal fats.

- Eat three pieces of fresh fruit and two portions of green and yellow vegetables daily.

- Include three portions of oily fish into your diet each week – mackerel, herring, pilchards, wild salmon or sardines.

- Go for a polyunsaturated spread rather than butter.

- Allow yourself one or two alcoholic drinks per day – it appears that red wine in particular may be good for the heart.

- Include in your diet garlic, onions, and some nuts, including walnuts, almonds and pecans.

- Regular exercise is a must.

- Indulge in formal relaxation at least 15–20 minutes each day.

- Take magnesium to lower high blood pressure as well as a strong B complex supplement. In addition 1 g of vitamin C per day as well as 200 mcg of the trace mineral chromium may also help to lower blood cholesterol levels.

- And, finally, there have been many positive studies on the beneficial properties of garlic – Kwai Garlic has been shown to reduce blood cholesterol, increases blood fluidity, lowers blood pressure and generally reduces the incidence of heart disease.

Depression

The word depression is used to describe such a wide range of moods, from the low spirits we all experience occasionally to a severe problem, that it is often misunderstood. It is much more than the bitter disappointment or deep sadness, which are temporary reactions to events such as the loss of a loved one or being turned down for a job. Although hard to bear, these are part of life and do eventually pass for most of us.

Depression, however, causes long-lasting changes in your mood, behaviour and feelings. You can't pull yourself together and a walk in the park or a weekend break won't solve the problem. It's a very real, debilitating condition that needs medical attention and treatment, and it will certainly be a barrier to feelings of well-being and weight loss. Depression is not something you can easily snap out of without help and left untreated can interfere with daily life and relationships. Once your GP has ruled out physical causes for your change of mood you should ask for referral for treatment such as counselling, cognitive behaviour therapy or psychotherapy, rather than prescribing medication. There are several alternative therapies and self-help tactics that can help to bring relief from depression and these should be the first choice for doctors.

CAUSES: Common triggers for depression include a major life event such as divorce, separation, long-term illness or job loss. An underactive thyroid can also produce symptoms of depression, as well as preventing the sufferer from being able to lose weight, and other serious illnesses such as cancer, kidney, liver or heart disease, anaemia and diabetes can also understandably cause depression. Sometimes depression appears to come from nowhere but it may be a delayed reaction to something that happened in your past. It can also be caused by changes in brain chemistry or by something in your genetic make-up.

Real life story

Jill Dunn was a retired teacher from Kent who lived with her husband and two sons. She was depressed and recovering from a nervous breakdown following extreme bullying she had experienced in the workplace, during which time she had gone up to a size 20.

❝ I took early retirement from work and felt like I was suffering with bereavement, grieving the loss of myself. I had terrible hot flushes and mood swings for which my doctor prescribed HRT. Almost immediately, I started gaining weight – 70 lb (32 kg) in all – and started getting headaches and what felt like constant PMS. I had wind, bloating and constipation and was obsessed with chocolate. I then went through a period of feeling suicidal. My life was out of control and I didn't feel like I could deal with or handle anything. I knew I had to put some balance back into my life and my friend made me arrange to see Maryon.

Maryon suggested I came off the HRT and put me on the Real Life Diet and an exercise programme, which I followed as best I could. Within six weeks I felt like a different person. As the months passed I felt happier and more positive than I had for years the weight started to fall off and I went down to a size 10. I felt so energised that I had the enthusiasm to spring clean my life. It left me feeling calm and happy and people I knew walked by me in the street as my physical appearance had changed so much. As you can imagine I continue with the Real Life Diet as it has been my lifeline. ❞

Help yourself

In the short term, the following may help alleviate your symptoms:

- Keep your blood-sugar levels evenly balanced, to help even out moods, energy and concentration, by having regular meals containing protein-rich and fibre-rich foods, and avoiding sugar, alcohol, caffeine and all refined foods.

- You may be tempted to drown your sorrows but the relief you feel will only be short term and too much alcohol can actually make you feel more depressed.

- Eat plenty of oily fish, as omega fatty acids, especially EPA, have been found in studies to be beneficial in alleviating depression.

- If you are feeling bad, try to tell someone how you feel. Remember, admitting to depression is part of the way forward. So don't suffer in silence – be proactive and share your feelings with friends or your GP.

- Exercise is essential for a healthy body and mind. Go outside even if it's only for a walk. Exercise also encourages the production of endorphins, the body's own feel-good hormones.

- Make the time to relax and give your mind a break. Reflexology, flotation and t'ai chi all have wonderful stress-relieving properties. Don't be afraid to try something new. For more, see Chapter 7, page 78.

- Sleep is the most natural way to recharge your batteries. If you can't get to sleep, try a natural remedy such as valerian or sip a cup of soothing camomile tea before going to bed.

- Research shows a link between depression and a deficiency in the vitamins and minerals that supply the nervous system. A multivitamin and mineral formula will ensure you don't run low on vital nutrients, while a B complex supplement and magnesium can help to improve your mood. Research also shows that herbal supplements such as St John's wort can be just as effective as conventional antidepressants for treating mild to moderate depression. Check with your GP first though, if you are taking other medication.

- Try a massage. Cedarwood, lime, neroli and bergamot oils are all uplifting.

- The following Bach Flower Remedies can be helpful: Mustard when you're depressed for no apparent reason; White Chestnut if worrying thoughts keep going round and round in your head; Wild Rose if you feel unmotivated and resigned; Gorse if you are pessimistic and see only negative outcomes.

Constant tiredness

We all feel tired from time to time. Overwork, family pressures and so on can soon take their toll on our natural energy levels, but if you find yourself waking up feeling more tired than when you went to bed on more than the odd occasion it's time to take stock and do something about it. Being overtired is likely to erode your resolve to eat healthily or follow any diet plan and that's when junk food gets guzzled instead of wholesome food. To add to this, those who are tired don't usually engage in regular exercise, which is essential to a healthy lifestyle.

CAUSES: There could be many factors at work. Your diet could be at fault, you could be under unacceptable stress, you may be depressed (see above), your iron levels may be low or you may simply be unfit. Your tiredness could be caused by an underlying physical illness such as heart, liver or kidney disease, or thyroid problems. If you suspect this may be the case, visit your doctor for tests. Those who have certain types of allergy, including eczema, asthma, nettle rash, migraine headaches and bowel problems, including irritable bowel syndrome, may experience fatigue. In one study, allergy to wheat protein was linked with increased complaints of fatigue, headaches and bowel problems.

Help yourself

- Eat plenty of foods that help to stimulate your metabolism. That means including plenty of wholesome foods such as brown rice, quinoa, polenta and buckwheat noodles, plus your five portions of fruit and veg a day.

- Cut down on sugary and refined foods. They may give you a quick energy boost but it will only be short lived and you'll be reaching for the biscuit tin again in next to no time.

- How you eat can be as important as what you eat. Research shows that eating like a child, little and often, results in an increase in energy levels.

- Make sure you take in enough fluid. Not drinking enough can also bring on feelings of fatigue. Our muscles are made up of 75 per cent water and the metabolism needs enough water to function properly. Increase the fluid in your diet with soups, smoothies, and plenty of fruit and vegetables, which contain mainly water. Good choices include: cucumber, melon, lemons, strawberries, oranges, apricots, pears, tomatoes, grapes, avocados, bananas, cherries, mangoes and kiwi fruit. You should aim to drink six to eight glasses of water a day, and more if you are active. Keep away from coffee and tea, which are stimulants. Go for herbal teas instead.

- A good night's sleep is essential if you are to function at optimum levels. To make sure you sleep soundly, try to go to bed around the same time each night. Before turning in spend some time winding down. Have a warm bath to which you have added some essential oils such as camomile, orange blossom and lavender. Listen to some soothing music or read a good book. Avoid exciting TV programmes or videos late at night. A cup of calming camomile or Night Time tea can also help to get you ready for sleep.

- Despite what you might think, as long as you are getting enough sleep, resting is the worst thing you can do if you feel tired as it slows down your metabolic rate. According to the experts the more energy you expend through exercise, the more energy you will have. You should aim for at least half an hour a day of some kind of sustained aerobic activity – anything that makes you feel slightly breathless and forces you to breathe more deeply, bringing freshly oxygenated blood to the brain which will wake you up and increase your energy levels. For more on exercise, see Chapter 5.

- A build-up of stress can result in a tired and weary body. Try to establish an even balance between work and play – that is so vitally important. But take care not to play too hard, as it will only wear you out! For more ways to keep stress at bay see Chapter 6, Learning to love yourself.

- Look to your iron levels. Iron deficiency, which is more common in vegetarian women with heavy periods, for example, causes anaemia in four per cent of adult women of child-bearing age in the UK, with a further ten per cent of women of child-bearing age having evidence of low iron stores, and this may explain why fatigue is more common among women. Mild fatigue in such women responds to iron supplementation, which shows how a mild or severe nutritional deficiency can be a cause of chronic fatigue.

FIFTEEN TOP FOODS FOR HEALTH

Experts rate the following foods as being generally full of health-giving properties, as well as being of particular benefit in specific conditions as mentioned above:

➤

- BROCCOLI Rich in antioxidants, vitamins, minerals and fibre, broccoli is said to lower the risk of bowel cancer and protect the immune system, as well as improving skin and mood. Its powerful anti-cancer properties are due to its high content of the phytochemical sulforaphane.

- GARLIC As a natural antibiotic, garlic is a great immune booster, protecting the body against infection. It also has detox properties and will help to keep your heart healthy thanks to a substance called allicin, which helps to reduce clotting, and will keep a check on cholesterol levels.

- KIWI FRUIT Containing almost twice as much vitamin C as an orange and more potassium than a banana, as well as a wealth of antioxidants, the kiwi is one of the most nutritionally rich fresh fruits.

- BANANAS Well known for their slow-releasing, energy-boosting fruit sugars, bananas also have relaxant properties thanks to the amino acid tryptophan, which has a sedative effect. They are also rich in potassium, which helps to lower blood pressure and relieve muscle cramps, as well as being a good source of fibre.

- TOMATOES Full of nutrients, especially a substance called lycopene, tomatoes are good for blasting free radicals. They are delicious raw but cooking increases the cancer-fighting power of lycopene. A recent Italian study showed that men who ate ten or more tomatoes a week reduced their risk of prostate cancer by as much as 35 per cent.

- OILY FISH Salmon, tuna or mackerel are a must in every diet. They are one of the richest sources of omega-3 essential fatty acids, which the body needs to function at its best. As

➤

well as being vital for a healthy brain and nervous system, they are needed for cardiovascular protection, hormone production and promoting healthy hair, skin and nails.

- ALMONDS As well as being one of the best non-meat sources of protein, almonds are full of the bone-building minerals calcium, magnesium, manganese and phosphorus. They are also a good source of fibre and vitamin E and so help to protect against disease-causing free radicals.

- COOKING OILS A supply of oils will give you a good supply of healthy fats without causing weight gain. Extra virgin olive oil will help to zap disease-causing free radicals, while walnut and rapeseed oils contain heart healthy omega-3 fatty acids. Wheatgerm and sunflower oils supply skin enhancing vitamin E, and sesame oil contains sesamin, which is good for regulating blood pressure and cholesterol levels.

- GINGER Rich in calcium, magnesium, phosphorus and potassium, ginger is a popular anti-spasmodic, which helps prevent nausea and improve circulation. It can help dispel menstrual cramps and makes a soothing tea, which can be especially good during convalescence.

- SOYA Soya beans and any products made from them, such as tofu, tempeh, miso, soya milk and soy sauce, are rich in phytoestrogens, plant substances that mimic human oestrogen and have been shown to be especially beneficial for menopausal women, helping to control symptoms as well as having a protective factor against heart disease and osteoporosis. It is also thought soya may help to boost memory by promoting and protecting nerve cell communication, as well as having a protective effect on the prostate.

➤

- HONEY Twice as sweet as sugar but at least ten times better for you, honey has been used to heal and energise for centuries. It has powerful anti-inflammatory, antiseptic and virus-fighting properties.

- SWEET POTATOES Delicious and easy to cook, sweet potatoes have one-and-a-half times the RDA of vitamin A , 50 per cent of the RDA of vitamin C, and good amounts of three essential minerals: calcium, magnesium and potassium.

- BEANS They have a little fat but lots of key nutrients, including the B vitamin folic acid, copper, zinc, magnesium and potassium. They are also a good source of protein (usually found in higher-fat foods), fibre and complex carbohydrates, which will give you long-lasting energy. Two servings a day of your favourite bean can help to lower blood cholesterol by as much as 27 per cent.

- WATERCRESS A natural antibiotic that can help relieve stomach upsets, respiratory problems and urinary tract infections. It includes 15 essential nutrients including vitamins A, C, E, folic acid and calcium. It is also brimming with natural anti-cancer compounds called isothiocyanates, as well as the antioxidant lutein, needed for healthy eyes.

- PUMPKIN SEEDS Rich in calcium, iron, magnesium and zinc, pumpkin seeds also contain omega-3 and omega-9 essential fatty acids. They are excellent for prostate health.

Which supplements?

The range of supplements is growing all the time and there is a huge array of products from which to choose. But if you are experiencing any of the symptoms mentioned in the questionnaires in this book, if you choose carefully your investment will certainly be repaid in terms of increased health. Here's our guide to help you make your choice.

- **General multivitamins and multi-minerals:** The better multivitamins have a good range of vitamins and sometimes minerals at a level close to the UK RDA (recommended daily allowance) or RNI (reference nutrient intake).

- **Multivitamins with iron:** These are similar to ordinary multivits, but contain additional iron, which is often required by women with heavy or prolonged periods.

- **Strong multivitamins:** These can contain 5–30 times the usual daily amount of some of the B vitamins, which can be particularly beneficial if your diet is on the poor side and especially if you like to drink alcohol, or you experience anxiety or depression.

- **Single supplements:** There is a wide variety of single supplements. Among the best known are iron, which is useful for heavy periods, and zinc, which helps with acne and poor healing, but there are a number of other single supplements that are worth a special mention here:

Calcium (as calcium carbonate, lactate or citrate) is useful as a preventive measure for anyone on a low calcium diet, for example, a dairy-free or vegan diet. A typical dosage is 300–600 mg daily. Calcium is best taken with meals but must

➤

not be taken with bran. Calcium helps prevent the bone-thinning disease osteoporosis (best combined with exercise and magnesium).

Magnesium (as oxide, citrate or chelate) supplements provide 100–150 mg per tablet. It is essential for nerve, hormone and muscle function. Intakes in the UK are acknowledged to be borderline or deficient in some 10 per cent or more of adults. In our own surveys of women with premenstrual syndrome (PMS), we have repeatedly found that over 50 per cent of women with PMS have low magnesium stores, indicating that magnesium can be useful for PMS. It is also useful for muscle cramps or constipation. Higher doses act effectively as a laxative.

Vitamin C, at doses of between 2–4 g per day, **zinc**, at doses of 30 mg per day, and **vitamin A** (as palmitate), at doses of 25,000 iu per day, can also help to boost the immune system if you are in a low state or suffering with a post-viral condition.

Evening primrose oil (quarma) can be helpful for eczema and premenstrual breast tenderness and period pain at 2–4,000 ius per day.

Marine fish oil (cardiozen) can be particularly good for helping skin problems such as dry skin and psoriasis, plus it can be helpful with painful periods and in preventing heart disease. Take 4–6 fish oil capsules at night.

Folic acid, at a dose of 400 mcg per day, should be taken by women who are trying to conceive, or who may fall pregnant, and it should be taken daily for four months before conception, through to the end of the first three months of pregnancy, as it has been shown to reduce the

➤

risk of birth defects such as spina bifida by as much as 70 per cent.

The **antioxidants vitamin A** (as betacarotene), natural **vitamin E** and **vitamin C** (with bioflavenoids), and the minerals **selenium, zinc, manganese** and **copper,** can help to protect against cancer and environmental toxins.

Optivite (only available by mail order; see below) is a **magnesium**-rich multivitamin and mineral supplement, designed for women of childbearing age, which has been through four properly conducted hospital trials and has been shown to improve premenstrual syndrome, and influence brain chemistry and hormone function positively.

Gynovite (available by mail order; see below) is a **magnesium**-rich multivitamin and mineral supplement, designed for women from the menopause onwards, which has been through two clinical trials and has been shown to help to correct nutrient levels in the body and help to improve bone density.

Health Insurance Plus (available by mail order; see below) is a strong multivitamin and mineral preparation that helps to promote nutritional balance in men.

The recommended supplements are available by mail order from the Natural Health Advisory Service (see Useful Addresses on page 328).

Herbal helpers

Some herbal supplements have been shown by clinical trials to be just as effective as drugs in helping to overcome certain symptoms. While vitamins and minerals can be taken in the long term, herbal preparations are usually best taken while addressing a particular problem. For example, the effects of a course of echinacea will last for anything from a few weeks to a month, and the recommended course for St John's wort is three months.

Here are a few examples:

- **St John's wort**, known as the sunshine supplement, has repeatedly been shown to help overcome depression and in Germany is more widely prescribed by doctors than the anti-depressant Prozac. It has also been shown to help combat seasonal affective disorder (SAD).

- **Ginseng** has been revered for thousands of years in China for its ability to boost energy and vitality. There is also evidence that it contains compounds with sex hormone activity, and studies have shown it may help overcome impotence caused by sex hormone deficiency.

- **Rhodiola**, a native herb of Siberia, has been shown to help beat stress. It is also an effective anti-depressant and has a reputation as an aphrodisiac, probably due to its ability to lift mood and improve stamina.

- **Butterbur, ginger** and **feverfew** have all been shown to relieve the symptoms of migraine headaches.

- **Novogen red clover,** a plant-based supplement, which contains isoflavones, has been shown in numerous clinical

➤

trials to help to control symptoms of the menopause including hot flushes, night sweats and vaginal dryness.

- **Echinacea** is a herb that is used to boost the immune system.

- **Valerian** helps to combat nervous tension and insomnia.

- **Passiflora** helps with anxiety, tension, irritability and sleeplessness.

- **Buchu** helps to relieve wind and bloating.

- **Artichoke** and **slippery elm** help to combat indigestion and soothe the gut.

- **Blue flag** helps with acne, boils and other skin infections.

- **Primula** helps to combat catarrh.

- **ArginMax** helps to improve libido.

- **Ginkgo Biloba** (120 mg of extract daily) helps to maintain circulation of the blood and maintain the bloods oxygen supply which helps to restore both short and long term memory.

- **Trinovin** is an isoflavone rich supplement – containing 40 mg of standardised isovlavones – which helps to maintain a normal healthy prostate.

- **Chromium Complex** (1 tablet a day) helps combat cravings for food, as it contains chromium, B vitamins and magnesium, which have all been shown to be necessary for normal blood glucose control.

- **Muira Puama** the Brazilian herb with aphrodisiac properties, is available in 2500 mg tablets by Rio Trading Company

➤

- **Damiana** (a 325 mg capsule) by Arkopharma, is also used as a natural aphrodisiac.

- **Arkopharma Phyto Soya Age Minimising Cream** has been shown to significantly decrease the depth of wrinkles and increase the firmness and thickness of the skin within a month.

- **Arkopharma Phyto Soya Body Firming Lotion,** which contains soya isoflavones, has been shown to help combat skin slackening and loss of skin density due to skin ageing.

- And, last but not least, **black cohosh** can help to relieve menstrual cramps and control hot flushes at the time of the menopause.

To order these supplements, or if you need some extra help in choosing the right supplements you can contact the NHAS for advice (contact details are on page 328).

Food for thought

Part One of this book should have opened your eyes to the possibility that there is work to be done on improving the balance in your body in an attempt to feel and look good as well as attain your target weight in the longer term. It's unrealistic to expect to coast through life feeling wonderful and sylphlike when there are chinks in the balance in some of the key departments of your life. It unfortunately isn't as simple as just improving your diet and achieving your target weight, because we know that most dieters regain the lost pounds within the space of a matter of months because of unaddressed issues. Making dietary changes helps, but there is much more to it. The feel-good factor comes as part of the package when you are eating well, and in addition keeping fit, not too stressed, depressed or tired, your relationships are satisfying, you have no backlogs at home or at work and you can look yourself in the eye with pleasure. And while that package might sound like a tall order, it is perfectly attainable.

I have lost count of the number of patients I have guided through the transformation over the years, from being overweight, depressed, lacking in energy and in many cases feeling overwhelmed by life, to feeling better than they can remember, with masses of energy, having lost weight and got back to a respectable level of fitness. And in each case it wasn't simply making dietary changes that achieved the objective, but rather us working together to restore the balance across the board in their lives. That's what gave them the key to losing weight, not only without dieting, but with the knowledge of how to remain in shape without regaining the lost pounds.

Now you've got the theory part under your belt, not forgetting the questionnaires filled in, you're ready to embark on the road to better health, well-being and weight loss – Stage 1 of the Real Life Diet!

Part Two

Maryon's Real Life Diet in Action

CHAPTER 11

The basic guidelines

The Real Life Diet is designed as a tool to help you find the right kind of diet for your body so that you can overcome unwanted symptoms and lose weight effortlessly. It is based on over 20 years of clinical experience and has proved to be a successful method of finding out what suits your needs both in the short and long term. If you have been a yo-yo dieter for years, the thought of starting yet another diet may give you that *déjà vu* feeling. This experience will be different though, for although it may seem unbelievable at this point, this is will be the last diet you are every likely to need. Not only will the Real Life Diet help you to shed your unwanted pounds, but a 'side-effect' of the programme is also health, well-being and balance, as a result of following the diet carefully over a period of several months. After the initial loss of fluid, which comes as a result of excluding foods that may cause a chemical reaction in the body and can sometimes be pretty dramatic in the first month, you are aiming for steady, gradual weight loss.

The aim of the Real Life Diet

As well as promoting weight loss, the Real Life Diet has been designed to fulfil a number of important criteria. It is:

- A balanced diet that will provide you with all the basic protein, carbohydrates, good fats and vitamins and minerals that your body actually needs to maintain optimum health.

- Rich in vitamins A, C and zinc, which all help to boost the immune system.

- Full of suggested menus that contain antioxidants, the vitamins and minerals that keep free radicals at bay, and help to prevent premature ageing and cancer.

- Designed to include those important essential fatty acids in the meal plans.

- Laden with suggestions of foods that contain phytoestrogens, which protect both men and women from all sorts of health problems.

The Real Life Diet is divided into three key stages. Stage 1, which lasts for four weeks, is the cleansing phase. This will help to give your body a rest and put back what time and nature have taken out. Stage 2, which lasts for four weeks, and Stage 3, lasting four weeks, will continue to give you all you need, while assessing whether your body can currently function well with certain food groups. In essence it is a ten-week plan, which can be extended if you decide it is necessary after reading the Real Life Extension (see page 220).

For each stage there are suggested menus and recipes to follow. As tastes and lifestyles differ the Real Life Diet has been designed to be accommodating. There are fast options for those who lead busy lives or simply dislike fussy cooking. If you like cooking, you may want to use the recipes provided in the recipe section beginning on page 224. If not, you can keep it simple and go for the easy options. For example, you can buy a tin of mixed beans instead of actually making the mixed bean salad, and smoothies made with soya milk are now available in the shops if you prefer to take a short cut. A comprehensive list of suggested breakfasts, lunches, dinners, snacks and beverages is given for each stage, together with sample menus for both omnivores (those who eat fish and meat) and also vegetarians. Provided you stick to the rules of each stage you can freely pick your menu from any of the sections. For example, one day you may prefer a fast option meal, another day a vegetarian meal, and perhaps at the weekend when you may have extra time to spend in the kitchen you could choose a more sophisticated menu. I have also included some additional recipes in the recipe section for you to try once you begin to feel more adventurous and want to add more variety into your regime.

In addition you can refer to the 'Nutritional content of food' lists that begin on page 299 and, with the exception of items that are off the menu of the current stage, you can choose the foods that you would like to include, knowing that they are full of good nutrients. This will help you to tailor the eating plan to your individual tastes, making it even more enjoyable.

What about calorie counting?

You can breathe a sigh of relief for we are not going to be counting calories, or weighing food. This does not mean that you can eat vast quantities of food at one sitting, especially if you need to lose weight, but instead eat slowly until you feel satisfied. This may seem amazing, bearing in mind that many diets do involve calorie counting, but the thousands of people who have successfully followed Stage 1 of the Real Life Diet over the years have not had to either weigh their food or count calories. If you remember I mentioned in Part One that finding the right plan for each individual seems to have a normalising effect on metabolism, which results in weight loss for those who are overweight.

I also suggest you weigh yourself once each week, first thing in the morning, without clothes, rather than obsessing about jumping on the scales each day.

Getting your facts straight

The Real Life Diet, unlike other diets, does not involve avoiding carbohydrates, which can be damaging to important organs in the body in the long term. Instead it provides a healthy balanced diet and is designed to help individuals to learn to get to know their bodies. It takes on board the principles of the Glycaemic Index (GI), a currently popular diet system, which has medical endorsement, but goes further as it allows the individual to undertake an experiment, which will ultimately teach them how to meet their own special nutritional needs, safely, both in the short and long term.

What is the Glycaemic Index?

GI has become a nutritional buzzword in the past few years. Indeed, Tesco, the UK's largest supermarket chain, have had 500 of their foods scored on the Glycaemic Index, but do you really know what GI refers to?

GI is a method of ranking foods that raise blood glucose and it has nothing to do with the carbohydrate content of the food. It assesses foods according to how quickly they can be digested and converted to glucose, your body's energy source. So foods like lentils and peanuts, which have thick cell walls, are much more difficult for digestive enzymes to break through, and this therefore lowers the GI. Foods with a high GI rating cause a rapid rise in blood-sugar levels, while those with a lower rating result in a steadier, more gradual rise.

Many people's diets are high in foods with a high GI rating, such as potatoes, white rice, refined breads, cereals, biscuits and sugary products. They all provide a quick surge of energy to the body but this peak is short lived and, as soon it subsides, the body usually starts to crave another high GI food for a repeat energy fix. This can trigger a cycle of energy peaks and troughs fuelled by high GI snacking, leading to overeating, loss of energy and weight gain.

The only way to break the cycle is to include more foods with a lower GI rating in your diet such as oats, pulses, fresh and dried fruits, which provide a more constant supply of energy. You can also combine some of high GI foods with other foods to reduce their GI rating. So, for example, combining pasta, which is has a high GI rating, with tomato sauce or tuna, will reduce its glycaemic index. The same happens when you combine a jacket potato with cheese and sweetcorn; and rice when combined with chicken curry.

Low GI foods are usually healthy foods and as they release energy more slowly they are thought to reduce the appetite. One study, conducted by researchers at Oxford Brookes University, showed that a group of schoolchildren, who were given a low GI breakfast, then went on to choose a lunch that contained 150 calories less than their counterparts who had a higher GI breakfast. So, in theory, consuming a low GI diet will help to avoid the yo-yo effect on energy levels throughout the day, ensuring you feel awake, alert and ready for anything. The evidence that consuming a low GI diet will automatically result in weight loss in humans has not been established, but researchers have found that rats that were fed a low GI diet halved their body weight within 17 weeks!

A diet that achieves a balance between high and low GI foods tends to be healthier not least because it prevents the cravings for fatty sugary foods that often arise when blood sugar levels fall. It will also leave you feeling fuller for longer so your appetite decreases.

Research also shows that low GI diets help to control diabetes by improving blood sugar and fat metabolism. They may also help to prevent the onset of Type 2 diabetes. A recent study from the Hammersmith Hospital, where they monitored glucose for 24 hours in diabetics who were put on a low GI diet, found a reduced insulin response.

Real life story

Businessman **Peter Spencer**, 52, travels a lot for work and found that his lifestyle had severely influenced his reflection in the mirror.

❜ Too much travel and too many business meals at which I inevitably drank too much alcohol meant the weight gradually crept on. I am quite tall, so I suppose I could carry the extra weight without it noticing so much, but eventually I put on four stone and to my eye I became unrecognisable.

Finally, after a party-packed week in Las Vegas I looked in the mirror and hated what I saw. I was determined to get back into shape. I started reading about diet and met Maryon. As well as changing to low GI foods, I decided to give up all alcohol initially for six months and began eating five servings of fruit each day, lots of vegetables, grains, small portions of meat, and I cut out dairy products including milk and cheese. I began running again regularly which I hadn't done for ages. I lost that four stone in six months.

The weight just fell off. I haven't put back on any weight in two years, despite eating very well. My self-esteem is so much higher and I notice I can cope with stress more easily now.

I feel fit and far healthier and have bundles of energy. People who meet me for the first time can't believe that I was ever anything but fit, healthy and in great shape which is just how I like it. ❞

How to read the GI

Pure glucose produces the largest rise in blood-sugar levels and has a reading of 100. All other foods are ranked from 0–100 according to their effect on blood-sugar levels.

High GI foods (70 or more) should make up less than 10 per cent of your diet

Medium GI foods (69–56) should make up 30 per cent of your diet

Low GI foods (55 or less) should make up 40 per cent of your diet

High GI foods: honey, potatoes, parsnips, bananas, butter, cheese, cream, full fat milk, wheat flakes, white bread, pasta and rice, pastries, biscuits and cakes, cashews, peanuts, pistachios, all processed foods, red meat, chocolate, tea, coffee and alcohol – but don't forget that combining them with other foods will lower their GI score, and consuming bananas that are slightly under-ripe will also have a much lower GI than the ripened fruit.

Medium GI foods: pineapple, mangos, apricots, raisins, skimmed or soya milk, wholemeal bread and pasta, brown rice, boiled potatoes, couscous, spaghetti, pitta bread, digestives and oat biscuits, sunflower and pumpkin seeds, taco shells, water biscuits and sweetcorn.

Low GI foods: apples, cherries, fresh dates and figs, limes, strawberries and pears, asparagus, aubergines, broccoli, cabbage, carrots, cauliflower, celery, courgettes, leeks, sweet potato, spinach, turnips, millet, quinoa, wild rice, butter beans, chickpeas, kidney beans, lentils and soya beans, almonds, brazil nuts, sesame seeds, fish oils, nut oils and avocado oil.

Healthy choices

The quality of our food is not always as Mother Nature intended, so our food choices are all important. The little extra time you spend planning your diet and shopping for healthy organic food where possible, and the little extra money it may cost will all pay dividends in the long term. And your healthy diet does not need to be any more expensive than your previous diet. If you think about what the average premenstrual woman might spend on chocolate, for instance, and what we spend on pre-prepared food and alcohol, there will be areas where you can undoubtedly make savings. A good start is to concentrate on buying fruit, salad and vegetables that are in season, rather than making exotic choices.

There are other Hot Tips that will help you achieve success in the Real Life Diet, and these will be looked at in the next chapter.

CHAPTER · **12**

Real Life Diet hot tips

Despite there being no calorie counting in the Real Life Diet, there are rules or Hot Tips, which do need to be followed in order to achieve success. If you have been battling with the bulge for some time you have, no doubt, often regarded yourself as your own worst enemy. Equally, you can be your own best friend by treating your eating habits and your lifestyle seriously. With the Real Life Diet it's not simply a matter of following a restricted diet; instead you will need to learn to pamper your body with the foods it likes, while working to keep yourself in good physical shape. The mental attitude and your lifestyle are just as important as the selections you take to the check-out at the supermarket. Initially, as with any new diet, there will be an element of willpower needed in order for you to adhere to the rules, and the following tips will help to boost your ability to achieve your goals.

The hot tips

- Make a start on the Real Life Diet when you have the time; ideally when you have a few clear weeks without any major commitments.

- It's important to get into the habit of completing your daily diary, which you will find on page 311, right away. The information recorded on the diaries will be useful to refer back to as you go along.

- You need to plan and set aside time for planning, shopping, preparation and consumption of meals.

- Rather than shopping weekly for all your food, it would be preferable to shop at least twice each week, especially for fruit, vegetables and salad stuff, as the shelf life of vitamins and minerals is quite short. Make sure you store fresh produce in the refrigerator or somewhere very cool to prevent them from spoiling.

- Go shopping before beginning your diet, preferably after you have eaten so that you are not starving hungry and tempted to cheat. Letting someone loose in a supermarket when they are both hungry and overweight should be a criminal offence!

- Make a shopping list as you plan your diet for the week and take it with you, making sure you stick to it.

- Eat regular meals, at least three meals a day, preferably with two small snacks in between if you feel hungry.

- Never miss a meal. Irregular eating leads to less healthy weight loss and increased feelings of hunger.

- It is useful to eat from a small plate not a large one. A well-stocked, medium-sized lunch or breakfast plate looks more satisfying than a large dinner plate only half filled.

- Chew your food well and savour each mouthful. Try not to hurry your meals.

- Eat fresh foods whenever possible. If at all possible, prepare one meal at a time. If this is not practical, try cooking a chicken, for example, to eat cold over a period of several days.

- Grill food rather than fry to keep your fat consumption low and to preserve the nutrients.

- Never eat a meal when you are in a hurry. Have a snack instead until you have the time to sit down to a proper meal. A good way to break the habit of eating too quickly is to put your knife and fork down after each mouthful.

- Make mealtimes special and enjoy your food. First, you should set aside time to prepare your meal. Always eat sitting down and only sit down to eat when everything is ready: the meal itself, drink, cutlery and the required condiments. Do not watch television while you are eating, but instead look at your food and savour it.

- Look again at Chapter 3, make a note of any particular require-ments you have for your current stage and incorporate those into your programme.

Decisions to live by

It is important to identify your personal reasons for wanting to be slimmer and feel healthier. Recent research has shown that people who list the consequences of dieting, positive and negative, and remind themselves of these consequences regularly during the day, do twice as well on their diets as those people do not do so. It is a good idea to list the positive and negative consequences of dieting on an index card, which you can then carry around and refer to prior to eating or exercising.

Below is an example of a chart that you could construct on a card or in your diary, with Immediate consequences on one side and Long-term consequences on the reverse. Give some thought to each column before listing the reasons why you want to lose weight. Complete it after eating – not before. Once your chart is complete, refer to it at least at mealtimes, and any other time you feel tempted to cheat!

Immediate consequences

	Positive	Negative
Following the Real Life Diet	Improved mood	Bother of getting educated
	Feeling of well-being	
	Self-satisfaction	Possible withdrawal symptoms
	Approval from friends and family	Changing old habits
	Weight loss	Having to change lifestyle
	Better relationships	Family eating habits change
	More energy	
	Improved appearance	Having to exercise
Continuing with the previous eating habits	No changes required	Poor self-image
	Short-term satisfaction	Feel bloated and overweight
	No expense on new clothes	Feel generally below par

Long-term consequences

	Positive	Negative
Following the Real Life Diet	Feeling of well-being	Restricted indulgences in some favourite foods and drinks
	Pleasing appearance	
	Sense of achievement	
	Improved health for all the family	
	Happier with self and life	
Continuing with previous eating habits	No effort required	Self-conscious of size
	Social satisfaction of 'free' eating	Feel uncomfortable and bloated
		Feel unwell
		Increased health risks
		Expense of larger clothes!

Having taken the tips on board and the time to reflect on your reasons for undertaking the Real Life Diet you are now ready to set out upon your voyage through Stage 1.

CHAPTER 13

What's on the menu?

Now let us look at what you can and can't eat during Stage 1 of the Real Life Diet. It is probably similar in many ways to diets you have seen or read about before, but there are some very important differences, which is why it is so successful.

Foods that can be eaten

In the first four weeks of the Real Life Diet, Stage 1, it is very important to eat only the allowed foods. If you introduce other foods you will lose the beneficial effects of the diet and it will be necessary for you to begin again.

Meat and poultry

For non-vegetarians: all meat, including lamb, beef, pork, chicken, turkey, other poultry and game, and offal such as liver, kidneys, sweetbreads and hearts, can be eaten if desired. Meat and poultry can be fresh or frozen.

Meat must be lean, with all visible fat trimmed before cooking.

Do not eat the skin of chicken or other poultry; it should be removed before or after cooking.

Fish and shellfish

For non-vegetarians: all types are included and they may be fresh or frozen. Do not eat the skin, as it is high in fat and calories.

Note: all meat, poultry and fish should be cooked by grilling, dry-roasting, steaming, baking or stir-frying with low-fat ingredients, eg tomatoes or vegetables.

All vegetables

You can and should eat large amounts of vegetables, especially green ones or salad foods daily. Your allowance will be detailed in the daily menus.

Root vegetables, eg potatoes and parsnips, are limited to one small portion per day if desired. Beans and peas, which are protein-rich vegetables, are also included in moderate amounts.

Vegetarian proteins

For vegetarians and vegans these are an essential part of the diet. You are allowed all types of nuts, beans, peas, lentils, seeds, corn (maize), rice and potatoes. Vegans in particular should have two or three portions of these per day. Some people experience abdominal bloating and wind with beans and these should be well cooked to minimise this effect.

Fruits

All fruits are allowed, except glacé fruits and tinned fruits with sugar. Keep tinned fruits without sugar, and dried fruits to a minimum. If you want to eat bananas (the world's most popular fruit), half of one is equal to a single fruit portion.

Your fruit allowance amounts to three pieces of fruit per day. Fruit can be eaten whole or as a fruit salad. There is a recipe for fruit salad on page 284.

Reduced calorie foods

Fortunately, there are now many excellent calorie-reduced versions of such foods as salad dressings, mayonnaise, soups and baked beans. As a rule pre-prepared meals should be avoided on the Real Life Diet.

Vegetable oils and vegetable mayonnaise

A small amount of these foods is allowed daily. You can have up to two teaspoons of a low-fat polyunsaturate-rich margarine, such as Flora Light, per day. There are no fried foods on the diet (you didn't really expect them, did you?), but there are some stir-fry dishes and here you just wipe the inside of the pan or wok with a piece of kitchen roll dipped in sunflower or corn oil.

Nuts and seeds

Brazil nuts, almonds, pistachios, cashews, peanuts, sunflower seeds and sesame seeds are very nutritious, but unfortunately high in calories. If you are eating Wake Up Muesli (see page 227 for recipe) for breakfast that will be considered to be your daily allowance of nuts, seeds and dried fruit. Wake Up Sprinkle (see page 227), which is made up of ground nuts and seeds, is allowed on three occasions during a week to help liven up a salad or a fruit dish.

Rice and other salads

White or brown rice of any variety – long grain, short grain or basmati – is allowed. It will often be used instead of potatoes. Rice cakes (a rice crispbread) can be used in place of bread, but will usually be combined with other foods to lower the GI score. For example, if you add nut butter to rice cakes and serve rice with meat or as a risotto with cheese and vegetables, you will lower the GI score of the rice. Additionally, buckwheat, which is part of the rhubarb family and not wheat as it suggests, polenta, bamboo shoots, sago and tapioca can be used from time to time, but these do not appeal to everyone's palate.

Breakfast cereals

Only corn flakes and rice cereal, and Wake Up Muesli (see page 227) are allowed in Stage 1. They contain a good amount of protein and are often fortified with extra vitamin B and iron. Other breakfast cereals are not permitted in the first stage.

Eggs

Up to seven eggs per weeks are allowed, unless you have a very high cholesterol level. They are highly nutritious and very good value for money.

Foods to be avoided or severely limited

Wheat, oats, barley and rye, millet and bran

All foods made with these are to be avoided, apart from the exceptions given below. This means no ordinary cakes, biscuits, puddings, pasta, pastry, pies, porridge, or breakfast cereals, apart from those mentioned in the lists above, but there are many acceptable alternatives. There are some cake, biscuit and pudding recipes to be found on pages 280–98 of this book. Bread made with wheat flour is off the menu until towards the end of Stage 2, but alternatives may be used. For example, see the Rice Bread or Cornbread recipe on page 232, or try one of the wide variety of wheat-free products now available in supermarkets, health food shops and from websites supplying by mail order (see page 320).

Dairy products

Milk, cream and cheese are off the menu at this stage. Use soya milk and yogurt, or rice milk, as substitutes in Stage 1. Butter or a polyunsaturated low-fat spread is allowed in very small quantities: one or two level teaspoonfuls per day. However, if you have premenstrual tension, painful breasts or an elevated blood cholesterol level, you should have a low-fat polyunsaturated spread instead of butter.

Foods containing milk, cream, cheese, milk solids, non-fat milk solids, lactalbumin, whey, caseinates and lactose should be avoided. The only exception is polyunsaturated margarine, which often contains a very small amount of milk protein, lactalbumin or whey.

Vegetarians, ie non-meat or fish eaters, should use soya milk fortified with calcium, and should consume either one egg per day or good portions of beans, peas, lentils and some nuts or seeds on most days.

Animal fats and some vegetable fats

Animal fats, some vegetable fats, hard margarine, lard, dripping and suet are out, as are palm oil and coconut oil, and foods containing them. Chemically, these vegetable oils are much more like saturated animal fats than good quality sunflower or corn oil, which are high in healthier polyunsaturates. Hard margarines made from hydrogenated vegetable oils are also off the menu.

Sugar, honey, glucose and fructose (fruit sugar)

Any food made with these should be avoided. This means cakes, biscuits, most ice cream, sweets of all kinds, chocolate and puddings. This is not as depressing as it sounds. You will find suggestions for low-calorie desserts for each evening of the diet.

Fruit juices are high in fructose, which weight for weight has the same calories as sucrose (ordinary sugar), so if you wish to include them water them down.

Alcohol

You name it – alcohol's out initially. Sorry! Don't do this diet over Christmas. Even low-calorie alcoholic drinks, though they are a great improvement, are still all too high in empty calories. You will, however, get the chance to reintroduce alcohol in Stage 2.

Yeast-rich foods

All yeast-rich foods are to be excluded initially and they include any foods containing yeast extract: Marmite, Oxo, Knorr and other stock cubes, vinegar and pickled food, chutneys, piccalilli, sauces, or condiments containing yeast extract or vinegar.

Salt

Salt should not be used in cooking or at the table. This is particularly true if you experience fluid retention or high blood pressure. Salty foods such as ham, bacon and any other salted meats should be eaten sparingly. Crisps, peanuts and many convenience meals should not be on the menu at all. If you really cannot do without salt, then use a potassium-rich salt substitute like LoSalt. Try flavouring any salads, vegetables or cooked main dishes with pepper or herbs instead of salt. You should find that your taste for salt reduces as you progress through the diet.

Caffeine and tannin

Both caffeine and tannin should be kept to an absolute minimum, or better still substituted with alternative drinks. Remember that caffeine can be found in coffee, tea, chocolate and cola, plus some over-the-counter drugs. Tannin is usually found in tea and red wine.

Try to have no more than two decaffeinated drinks per day, as these contain other chemicals, and instead use alternatives like dandelion coffee, particularly ground root rather than instant, Rooibosch, or Redbush, tea, which is a good tea 'lookalike', chicory or any of the herbal teas.

Foods with additives

These cannot be avoided completely, but it is best to avoid those with some types of colouring and preservatives as they can cause asthma, nettle rash (urticaria), eczema and possibly migraine.

Avoid the following additives where possible:

E102	Tartrazine
E104	Quinoline Yellow
E110	Sunset Yellow FCF or Orange Yellow
E122	Carmoisine or Azorubine
E123	Amaranth
E124	Ponceau 4R or Cochineal Red A
E127	Erythrosine BS
E131	Patent Blue V
E132	Indigo Carmine or Indigotine
E142	Green S or Acid Brilliant Green BS or Lissamine Green
E151	Black PN or Brilliant Black PN
E180	Pigment Rubine or Lithol Rubine BK
E220–227	Sulphites – these may worsen asthma in very sensitive individuals

Other colourings are not likely to cause any adverse reactions.

Suspect foods

Avoid any foods that you know do not suit you. For example, many people find some fruits, such as oranges or pineapple, too acidic. Even though they are not particularly high in calories you should avoid them. A not infrequent problem is an inability to digest beans, peas and some vegetables properly, resulting in excessive wind. Possible vegetables in this group include cabbage, cauliflower, onions and sweetcorn. At this point, trust your 'sixth sense' and 'gut' feelings. After all, it is this sense that we want to increase, so let's not go against anything you know already, even if it means adapting the menus to suit your needs.

Modifications for vegetarians

Vegetarians and vegans should also allow peas, beans, lentils, soya milk, non-fermented soya produce, and increased amounts of nuts, seeds and rice. Sample vegetarian menus for Stage 1 begin on page 183.

CHAPTER 14

Real Life Diet – stage 1

You now have the tools to work out your nutritional requirements, and an exercise and relaxation programme to suit your schedule. It is now time to move on so that you can get started on Stage 1 of the Plan. You will need to fill in your weekly report forms (see page 309), allowing you to make a note of everything that crosses your lips, plus details about the exercise you successfully undertake, time spent relaxing and your supplement intake. Take care to complete these each day as they will prove to be an excellent source of referral as you progress through the three stages of the diet.

The first week of the diet plan is usually the hardest part to get through, as it is likely that you will experience withdrawal symptoms, especially if you have been a regular caffeine consumer.

Warning: If you persevere with the Real Life Diet the benefits are likely to be great!

Making a start

What can I expect?

The idea of excluding foods in this section is to give your body the chance to feed back to you whether certain food groups are causing symptoms and preventing you from losing weight in the short term. This often happens when nutrient levels are low, as the brain chemistry and subsequently the immune system cannot function normally, usually resulting in weight gain as well as a sense of lack of well-being. You will probably notice during the beginning of Stage 1 that you experience some withdrawal symptoms as a direct result of giving up certain foods and drinks that you usually consume. These symptoms may be anything from headaches to fatigue or even depression, and can last for anything from a few days to a week.

The degree to which you suffer will depend on your existing diet. For example, if you are consuming lots of cups of coffee or tea, cola drinks or refined sweet foods, you may find the first week of the diet is quite a challenge! Unfortunately there is no magic button to press that will get you through this phase completely unscathed, but cutting down gradually over a period of days or even a couple of weeks does seem to lessen the pain if you have been a heavy consumer.

It is probably best to begin the diet when you have a quiet week to spare. Women should begin the diet just after their period has arrived and not in the week their period is due in order to prevent additional symptoms occurring at a time when they might be feeling vulnerable.

You will need the time to accustom yourself to your new way of eating and to get plenty of relaxation. This doesn't mean that you should take time off work; quite the opposite, as it is preferable that you remain occupied while on the diet. Just keep social arrangements that involve eating to a minimum. Then, if you feel tired or experience any withdrawal symptoms, you can go off to rest without any guilty feelings.

Your individual needs

As you worked your way through the questionnaires in Part One of the Real Life Diet you will have compiled lists of your personal requirements. So, in addition to the general instructions given in Stages 1, 2 and 3, you will need to incorporate your own personal needs into your regime. So, if you are supposed to be including soya into your diet two or three times a day, or taking specific nutritional supplements and getting some daily relaxation and exercise, you will need to include these recommendations in your regime in order to maximise your success in both the weight loss and the well-being departments.

Daily diaries

Diaries are provided in the appendix (pages 309–12) to give you the opportunity to record all foods, drinks and supplements that pass your lips each day, together with any exercise and relaxation that you undertake. In addition, you have space in the diary to record any symptoms you experience, ranging from withdrawal symptoms to food and drinks in the first few weeks of the Real Life Diet, to adverse symptoms you may experience when introducing new food groups to your regime as you progress. While the prospect of daily admin may seem like hard work, research over a number of years has shown that the effort will pay dividends. Being faced with the prospect of maintaining a daily diary will undoubtedly 'encourage' you to follow the rules to the letter, and even to go the extra mile on the exercise and relaxation, perhaps at a time when you might otherwise turn over and go back to sleep. Once you have established your Real Life Diet, and begin to experience the benefits, it will become easier. The records become increasingly important in Stage 2 and in the longer term, when reintroducing foods and drinks that have been omitted from your diet for several weeks. They provide an ongoing record, essential to the efficient monitoring of your progress.

After the first week or so of following the diet, with any possible withdrawal symptoms behind you, things should look up. By Week 3, you should have lost a few pounds – at least four, possibly as many as eight – and you may notice that a number of minor health problems have begun to improve. By Week 4, you should be feeling quite well; perhaps better than you have felt for some time and, with any luck, you will be a good deal nearer to your target weight. It is important to continue with Stage 1 until any symptoms you have been suffering, such as fatigue, anxiety, bowel problems or headaches, have abated. This will allow you to attribute any symptoms you experience in Stage 2 to the foods you are introducing rather than your chronic health state.

FOCUS ON WEEK 1

The first week of any healthy eating campaign is usually the worst as you are likely to experience withdrawal symptoms to some of the foods and drinks you have eliminated. Expect to feel out of sorts for a few days. You may feel irritable, restless and uptight, and could even suffer headaches. The symptoms will pass in a matter of days and will be replaced by an ever-increasing sense of well-being.

Make a start on your new diet plan when you have sufficient time to commit to it, ideally when you have a few clear weeks without any major commitments, and make sure you set aside time for planning, shopping and food preparation.

This first week is **free from** wheat, oats, rye, barley and dairy products (including yogurt and goats' products). So 'alternative toast' refers to toasted bread free from wheat, oats, barley and rye. Also, 'homestyle' soup refers to any fresh soups available – such as the Covent Garden range.

> ## Remember. . .
>
> - You may experience withdrawal symptoms at first
> - Leave enough time for planning, shopping and food preparation
> - No wheat, oats, rye, barley or dairy

Now it's time to look at what you can eat during this week.
(* = see recipe in Chapter 17)

BREAKFASTS

- Wake Up Muesli* with soya milk/rice milk/soya yogurt
- Wake Up Yogurt Shake* with 2 tablespoons of Wake Up Sprinkle* blended in
- Fruit salad with Wake Up Sprinkle* and soya yogurt
- Gluten-free Pancakes* with pure stewed apple and soya yogurt
- Rice Krispies with a chopped banana and soya or rice milk
- Corn flakes with chopped almonds and soya or rice milk
- Boiled egg with rice cakes/corn crispbread or alternative soldiers
- Scrambled eggs, mushrooms and tomatoes with rice cakes/corn crispbread or alternative soldiers
- Mixed berry smoothie (mixed beans and soy milk blended with ice)

LUNCHES

- Beans on alternative toast
- Hummus with raw vegetable crudités and corn wafers
- Jacket potato with baked beans
- Jacket potato with tuna and salad
- Mixed bean salad
- Omelette

- Scrambled or poached eggs on alternative toast
- Rice salad with fish or chicken
- Home-made or 'homestyle' fresh soup

DINNERS

- Cold meat or fish with a large salad (see below)
- Corn pasta with Quorn or tofu in a tomato sauce with fresh herbs
- Corn tacos with mince or beans, guacamole and salsa
- Grilled gammon and pineapple and vegetables
- Cold chicken breast with a large salad and potato wedges or new potatoes
- Poached salmon with broccoli, carrots, sweetcorn and new potatoes
- Chicken and vegetable kebabs served with brown rice, sweetcorn and mangetout
- Prawn, chicken, Quorn or tofu stir-fry with rice noodles or brown rice

Salads should consist of salad leaves, rocket, baby spinach, watercress, tomatoes, cucumber and raw carrot. You can choose from a wide selection of salad leaves in the supermarket for convenience. Optional ingredients are peppers and spring onions added according to taste.

VEGETARIAN OPTIONS

- Mixed beans in tomato sauce with brown rice
- Spinach and mushroom omelette with a large salad
- Gluten-/dairy-free vegetarian sausages with baked beans and a jacket potato
- Quorn and vegetable kebabs served with brown rice, sweetcorn and mangetout
- Mexican Omelette* served with a large salad

- Corn spaghetti with a tomato and basil sauce with a few toasted pine nuts
- Quorn or tofu stir-fry with vegetables and brown rice or rice noodles

DESSERTS

- Stewed apple with home-made soya custard
- Stewed mixed berries (strawberries, blackberries, blueberries, raspberries) with soya yogurt
- Baked Apples*
- Meringue with Fresh Fruit Salad*
- Dried Fruit Compote*
- 'Swedish Glace' soya ice cream (available from some supermarkets and health food shops)
- Fruit Snow*
- Fresh fruit salad*

SWEET SNACKS

- Soya yogurt
- Soya fruit smoothie
- Dried fruit
- Fresh fruit
- Sesame seed bar
- Fruit strips
- Gluten-/dairy-free scone with pure fruit spread

SAVOURY SNACKS

- Raw vegetables
- Small amounts of unsalted nuts and seeds
- Rice cakes, corn crispbreads or 'Glutano' crackers with sugar-free fruit spread
- Japanese rice crackers
- Kettle crisps
- Mini poppadums

WEEK 1 SUGGESTED MENUS

DAY 1

BREAKFAST
Wake Up Muesli* with chopped fresh fruit and soya milk

LUNCH
Turkey breast with salad and a jacket potato

DINNER
Grilled mackerel or sardines marinated in lemon juice and black pepper with broccoli, mangetout and carrots

DESSERT
Baked Apples* with soya cream

DAY 2

BREAKFAST
Fresh Fruit Salad* with Wake Up Sprinkle* and soya yogurt

LUNCH
Scrambled eggs and baked beans on alternative toast

DINNER
Grilled chicken brushed with balsamic vinegar, honey and lemon juice, with brown rice, spinach and cauliflower

DESSERT
Stewed mixed berries (strawberries, blackberries, blueberries, raspberries) with soya yogurt

---

DAY 3

BREAKFAST
One boiled egg with 2 corn crispbreads or rice cakes

LUNCH
Jacket potato with baked beans and coleslaw salad

DINNER
Mixed Vegetable and Almond Stir-fry*

DESSERT
Meringue with fresh fruit salad

DAY 4

BREAKFAST
Gluten-free Pancakes* with fruit filling and soya yogurt

LUNCH
Home-made or 'homestyle' fresh soup with rice or corn cakes

DINNER
Grilled sardines with watercress, fennel and lemon salad

DESSERT
Swedish Glace soya ice cream

DAY 5

BREAKFAST
Puffed rice with chopped fresh fruit and nuts and soya milk

LUNCH
Spinach and mushroom omelette with a large salad

DINNER
Chicken and vegetable kebabs served with brown rice, sweetcorn and mangetout

DESSERT
Soya rice pudding with a spoonful of pure fruit spread

DAY 6

BREAKFAST
Two poached eggs with grilled tomatoes, plus two rice cakes or corn crispbreads

LUNCH
Beans on alternative toast with Green Salad*

DINNER
Corn tacos with mince or beans, guacamole and salsa

DESSERT
Mixed berry smoothie

DAY 7

BREAKFAST
Wake Up Muesli* with soya milk or rice milk plus a chopped banana

LUNCH
Raw vegetable crudités with corn chips and hummus

DINNER
Poached salmon with broccoli, carrots, sweetcorn and new potatoes

DESSERT
Fresh fruit salad with soya yogurt and a few chopped almonds

FOCUS ON WEEK 2

Now you should be over the worst! The withdrawal symptoms should have gone, or at least be calming down, and you should be feeling that there is a light at the end of the tunnel.

Have you been so absorbed with sorting yourself out for the first week, and coping with the withdrawal symptoms, that you forgot to check to see whether you have lost any weight? There are no hard and fast rules about how much weight you lose and how fast; it really does vary. For example, some individuals may lose large amounts of fluids at first, which registers on the scales as rapid weight loss. Other people may be slow and steady weight losers. Either way, it is important that you continue to feel well once the withdrawal symptoms have passed, and continue to satisfy the nutritional needs of your body.

In order to keep your diet interesting, and prevent boredom setting in, it would be advisable to track down some special foods for this stage of the Real Life Diet. Avoiding common ingredients in your diet, particularly wheat, which is found so commonly in foods, can be difficult unless you stock up with plenty of interesting and tasty alternatives. There are several varieties of acceptable rice, soya and corn breads, plus crackers, crisp breads, pastas and flour mixes available. The major supermarkets all have a wheat-free and an organic section these days and it is worth looking at some of the specialist health food shops for a wider range of delicious alternative products.

Don't just stick to rice cakes, but go on a 'shop crawl' to check out what the different local supermarkets and health food shops have to offer.

Never do your food shopping on an empty stomach. Take time to plan your diet for the coming week and make a shopping list. Take the list with you and make sure you stick to it! If possible, while you are adjusting to the Real Life Diet, it would be a good idea to set aside a little extra time at first for meal planning, shopping and food preparation. If you are short of time or lacking in energy, go for fast options, which require little or no cooking. It is easy to consume raw vegetable crudités and mini poppadums or corn chips, with dips like hummus or guacamole, or a serving of roast chicken with salad, which can all be bought pre-prepared.

Don't forget to keep a note of what you eat each day and how you feel in your diary so that you can look back through your records at the end of Stage 1.

You may be feeling pleased that you have lost a few pounds in the first week, but don't expect to lose weight as quickly every week. It is far better to follow a healthy eating plan and lose weight gradually while meeting your body's nutritional needs, since this way it is less likely that you will regain the weight at the end of the Plan.

Remember. . .

- Shop for interesting food alternatives
- Keep notes of your eating habits and feelings in your diary

---

Now it's time to look at what you can eat this week.
(* = see recipe in Chapter 17)

BREAKFASTS

- Wake Up Muesli* with soya milk or rice milk
- Corn flakes with Wake Up Sprinkle*, raisins and chopped nuts
- Corn flakes with a chopped banana and soya milk
- Gluten-free Pancakes* with maple syrup and chopped almonds
- Scrambled eggs, grilled mushrooms and tomatoes with rice cakes
- Veggie sausages (gluten/dairy free), grilled with mushrooms, tomatoes and rice cakes
- Alternative toast with nut butter
- Strawberry and banana smoothie

LUNCHES

- Grilled peppers, red onions, courgettes, baby plum tomatoes with balsamic vinegar and olive oil
- Chicken and apricot kebabs with salad
- Hummus with raw vegetable crudités and corn crackers

- Mackerel in olive oil with salad and a jacket potato
- Spinach omelette with salad
- Home-made or 'homestyle' soup with rice cakes or alternative toast

DINNERS

- Spanish Rice*
- Tofu/Quorn and vegetable stir-fry with rice noodles or brown rice
- Roast chicken (skin removed) with fresh vegetables and new potatoes
- Cold chicken or turkey salad with new potatoes
- Steamed cod with broccoli, mangetout and new potatoes
- Corn tacos with mince or beans, guacamole and salsa
- Mushroom and herb risotto
- Grilled salmon steak brushed with tamari sauce (wheat-free soya sauce), honey and lemon juice served with grilled courgettes, peppers and plum tomatoes
- Turkey and Chickpeas with Rice*
- Lamb chop with broccoli, mangetout, carrots and new potatoes

DESSERTS

- Fruit Snow*
- Baked bananas with cinnamon and ginger served with soya ice cream
- Stewed summer berries with soya yogurt
- Gluten-free Pancakes* with stewed plums and soya cream
- Fresh Fruit Salad*
- Swedish Glace soya ice cream
- Grilled nectarines sprinkled with a little brown sugar and crushed almonds

SWEET SNACKS

- Fresh fruit
- Organic dried fruit
- Soya yogurt
- Sesame seed bar
- Fruit strips
- Gluten-/dairy-free scone with pure fruit spread

SAVOURY SNACKS

- Rice cakes/corn cakes with pure fruit spread/nut butter
- Small amount of unsalted nuts and seeds
- Flavoured rice cakes
- Kettle crisps
- Mini poppadums

WEEK 2 SUGGESTED MENUS

DAY 1

BREAKFAST
Veggie sausages (gluten/dairy free), grilled with mushrooms, tomatoes and rice cakes

LUNCH
Home-made or 'homestyle' soup with rice cakes or alternative toast

DINNER
Steamed cod with broccoli, mangetout and new potatoes

DESSERT
Grilled nectarines sprinkled with a little brown sugar and crushed almonds

DAY 2

BREAKFAST
Corn flakes with Wake Up Sprinkle*, raisins and chopped nuts

LUNCH
Chicken and apricot kebabs with salad

DINNER
Spanish Rice*

DESSERT
Fresh Fruit Salad*

DAY 3

BREAKFAST
Gluten-free Pancakes* with maple syrup and chopped almonds

LUNCH
Mackerel with lemon stuffing*

DINNER
Roast chicken (skin removed) with fresh vegetables and new potatoes

DESSERT
Fruit Snow*

DAY 4

BREAKFAST
Strawberry and banana smoothie
Alternative toast with nut butter

LUNCH
Hummus with raw vegetables and corn crackers

DINNER
Grilled salmon steak brushed with tamari sauce, honey and lemon juice served with grilled courgettes, peppers and plum tomatoes

DESSERT
Swedish Glace soya ice cream

DAY 5

BREAKFAST
Wake Up Muesli* with soya milk or rice milk

LUNCH
Grilled peppers, red onions, courgettes, baby plum tomatoes with balsamic vinegar and olive oil

DINNER
Turkey and Chickpeas with Rice*

DESSERT
Baked bananas with cinnamon and ginger served with soya ice cream

---

DAY 6

BREAKFAST
Rice Krispies with a banana and a few almonds and sunflower seeds with soya or rice milk

LUNCH
Jacket potato with baked beans and salad

DINNER
Lamb chop with broccoli, mangetout, carrots and new potatoes

DESSERT
Soya yogurt with mango and strawberries

DAY 7

BREAKFAST
Two poached eggs on alternative toast with grilled tomatoes

LUNCH
Rice and nut salad

DINNER
Grilled fresh tuna steak marinated in lemon juice, garlic and tamari sauce, served with salad and new potatoes roasted in olive oil, rock salt and garlic

DESSERT
Rice pudding made with soya milk, served with pure fruit spread

FOCUS ON WEEK 3

By now you should feel that your energy levels are slowly returning. Some people come to this realisation gradually, while others just wake up feeling different one day. However this happens, it often feels like a great weight has been lifted from your shoulders.

Once you have your shopping sorted and your new eating plan established, you must invest your new-found energy wisely. A regular exercise routine will pay dividends in terms of providing both increased energy and rate of weight loss. Exercising four or five times each week, to the point of breathlessness, will stimulate your brain chemistry, making you feel so much better, plus it speeds up your metabolic rate, increasing the rate at which the body burns fat. Increase your pace gradually if you aren't used to exercising, remembering that it is not a competition, but you as an individual working to get your body into better shape.

If you haven't been very adventurous with your diet, through lack of time or motivation, make a point of introducing a few new products into your eating plan this week. Vary your snacks, perhaps prepare some wheat-free pancakes and add in some of the delicious sugar-free jams or spreads listed in the Healthy shopping options (page 311), especially if you are experiencing cravings for sweet food.

Making the time for quiet thought and reflection is also an important aspect of the programme, especially if you spend your time rushing around after others. Regular relaxation has been shown to decrease stress levels. If you are not familiar with yoga or meditation relaxation techniques, try the creative visualisation outlined in Chapter 7, which is both easy and immensely enjoyable.

Give yourself a pat on the back this week. You are now well on your way. It is so important to validate yourself for your efforts on a regular basis, rather than giving yourself a hard time mentally because you are still overweight and out of shape. Remember that Rome wasn't built in a day!

Remember. . .

- Establish an exercise routine that suits you

- Introduce new foods to keep the eating plan interesting

- Find time to relax

Now it's time to look at what you can eat this week.
(* = see recipe in Chapter 17)

BREAKFASTS

- Wake Up Muesli* with soya milk or rice milk
- Fresh Fruit Salad* with soya yogurt and 1 tbsp sunflower seeds
- Gluten-free Pancakes* with stewed apple and cinnamon
- Dried Fruit Compote* with soya yogurt (also a dessert)
- Banana and Mixed Summer Berry Smoothie* (also a dessert)

- Two poached eggs on alternative toast with grilled mushrooms and tomatoes
- Rice Krispies plus a chopped pear with soya milk
- Rice cakes with organic nut butter/pure fruit spread

LUNCHES

- Jacket potato with baked beans
- Mushroom omelette with salad
- Poached haddock, new potatoes and salad
- Home-made vegetable soup with rice cakes
- Stir-fried baby spinach, mangetout, pepper and courgettes with brown rice
- Hard-boiled egg salad with rice cakes
- Tinned sardines/mackerel and salad with rice cakes
- Soya yogurt with a chopped banana and some nuts and seeds
- Baked beans on alternative toast

DINNERS

- Chilli and Corn Fritters with Scrambled Eggs*
- Turkey and Chickpeas with Rice*
- Grilled chicken with lemon and black pepper served with assorted vegetables
- Oven-roasted Mediterranean vegetables (with chicken)
- Fresh tuna steak marinated in tamari sauce and lime served with salad
- Poached cod with spinach, broccoli, cauliflower and new potatoes
- Cold chicken, jacket potato and a large salad
- Green Chicken Curry*
- Vegetable Curry*
- Gluten-/dairy-free veggie burgers with coleslaw, potato wedges and salad

DESSERTS

- Soya yogurt with a few almonds
- Stewed apple, apricots and cinnamon with soya cream
- Banana and Tofu Cream*
- Mixed Summer Berry Smoothie*
- Meringue with fresh raspberries and soya cream
- Grilled fresh pineapple sprinkled with a little brown sugar
- Fresh fruit

SWEET SNACKS

- Fresh fruit
- Organic dried fruit
- Soya yogurt
- Sesame seed bar
- Fruit strips
- Gluten-/dairy-free scone with pure fruit spread

SAVOURY SNACKS

- Rice cakes/corn cakes with tahini or nut butter
- Small amount of unsalted nuts and seeds
- Japanese rice crackers
- Flavoured rice cakes
- Mini poppadums

WEEK 3 SUGGESTED MENUS

DAY 1

BREAKFAST
Wake Up Muesli* with chopped fresh fruit and soya milk

LUNCH
Turkey breast with Oriental Rice Salad*

DINNER
Stuffed Mackerel* with broccoli, mangetout and carrots

DESSERT
Gooseberry Jelly*

DAY 2

BREAKFAST
Fresh Fruit Salad* with Wake Up Sprinkle* and soya yogurt

LUNCH
Grilled sardines with Watercress, Fennel and Lemon Salad*

DINNER
Cumin Chicken* with brown rice, spinach and cauliflower

DESSERT
Baked Apples*

DAY 3

BREAKFAST
One boiled egg with two corn crispbreads or rice cakes with a scraping of polyunsaturated spread on each

LUNCH
Jacket potato with baked beans

DINNER
Mixed Vegetable and Almond Stir-fry*

DESSERT
Fruit Snow*

DAY 4

BREAKFAST
Corn and Rice Pancakes* with Dried Fruit Compote* filling and soya yogurt

LUNCH
Nut and Vegetable Loaf* with Courgette and Cauliflower Salad*

DINNER
Halibut Fruit* with braised fennel, mangetout and new potatoes

DESSERT
Banana and Tofu Cream*

DAY 5

BREAKFAST
Puffed rice with chopped fresh fruit and nuts, and soya milk or yogurt

LUNCH
Tomato soup with Cornbread* and Fruity Cabbage Salad*

DINNER
Chicken with Peach Sauce* served with potatoes and vegetables of your choice

DESSERT
Apple and Passion Fruit Delight*

DAY 6

BREAKFAST
Two poached eggs with grilled tomatoes, rice cakes and corn crisp breads with a scraping of polyunsaturated spread

LUNCH
Beans on alternative toast with Green Salad*

DINNER
Polenta with Grilled Vegetables*

DESSERT
Cranberry Sorbet*

DAY 7

BREAKFAST
Two slices of alternative toast with organic nut butter

LUNCH
Raw vegetable crudités with corn chips and hummus

DINNER
Hot Fruity Chicken* with carrots, spinach and jacket potato

DESSERT
Jellied Grapefruit*

FOCUS ON WEEK 4

Your efforts should really be paying dividends by now. The fourth week of Stage 1 of the Real Life Diet is often the time when you begin to feel really well and energised. The withdrawal symptoms of the first week or two have passed, as have the effects of your old diet on your body. If you felt sluggish before you began, or experienced a variety of common symptoms including headaches, mood swings or bowel problems, you should notice a general improvement. For persistent, or severe to moderate symptoms, diet alone may not be sufficient. It may be that you need the help of some specialist supplements to restore the nutrient balance in your body and keep the weight-loss procedure going. You will have a good idea whether or not you have nutritional deficiencies after completing the questionnaire 'Is your diet good for you?' If there is a deficiency, it is important that it is corrected by appropriate nutritional supplementation as well as a consuming a wholesome diet. For more on this, see page 124.

If you need to lose more than 10 lb (4.5 kg) in weight, but are otherwise in good health you are probably well advised to take a multivitamin and multi-mineral supplement. If in doubt a comprehensive multivitamin (with added iron, particularly if you are female and have heavy periods) is probably the best.

Remember that no special supplement of vitamins, minerals, or anything else for that matter, will melt your excess weight away. There is no substitute for a well-balanced, carefully selected diet, in which you take care to have an adequate intake of essential nutrients.

During your fourth week on the Real Life Diet you may find that your metabolic rate slows down as your body becomes used to the new way of eating and the reduced calorie intake. An excellent way of speeding up your metabolic rate again is to exercise four or five times each week to the point of breathlessness, increasing the intensity of your effort. You can choose any exercise you like, from brisk walking, a formal workout, swimming, racquet sports or even just dancing to your favourite music. Apart from helping to burn up the fat and tone your body, regular exercise results in an incredible sense of well-being and as an added bonus promotes long-term health.

Rather than shopping once a week for all your food, it is preferable to buy produce at least twice each week, especially fruit, vegetables and salads, as the shelf-life of the vitamins and minerals in them is quite short. Make sure you store fresh produce in the refrigerator or somewhere very cool, to prevent them from spoiling.

> ## Remember. . .
>
> - Consider whether you need to take supplements
> - Exercise four or five times a week
> - Shop for fruit, vegetables and salad at least twice a week

Now it's time to look at what you can eat during this week.
(* = see recipe in Chapter 17)

BREAKFASTS

- Wake Up Muesli* with soya milk or rice milk
- Rice Krispies with raisins and chopped nuts
- Gluten-free Pancakes* with stewed mixed berries
- Rice flakes and organic raisins soaked overnight in soya milk/apple juice with grated ginger, apple and cinnamon
- Corn flakes with a chopped banana and soya milk
- Scrambled eggs, grilled mushrooms and tomatoes with rice cakes
- Alternative toast with pure fruit spread
- Banana and Mixed Summer Berry Smoothie*

LUNCHES

- Grilled peppers, red onions, courgettes, baby plum tomatoes with balsamic vinegar and olive oil
- Scrambled eggs on alternative toast
- Chicken kebabs with salad
- Jacket potato with hummus and salad
- Grilled sardines with lemon juice, garlic and black pepper with salad
- Spinach omelette with salad

- Home-made or 'homestyle' with rice cakes or alternative toast
- Prawns marinated in lime, coriander and black pepper with salad

DINNERS

- Steamed salmon with broccoli, mangetout and new potatoes
- Salmon Steak with Ginger*
- Spanish Rice*
- Tofu/chicken and vegetable stir-fry with rice noodles or brown rice
- Spanish omelette with salad
- Roast chicken (skin removed) with fresh vegetables
- Cold chicken or ham salad with new potatoes
- Turkey, sweet potato and spinach curry with brown rice
- Corn tacos with mince or beans, guacamole and salsa
- Hard-boiled egg salad with a jacket potato
- Grilled salmon steak brushed with tamari sauce, honey and lemon juice served with grilled courgettes, peppers and plum tomatoes
- Turkey and Chickpeas with Rice*

DESSERTS

- Fruit Snow*
- Baked bananas with cinnamon and ginger served with soya ice cream
- Stewed summer berries with soya yogurt
- Gluten-free Pancakes* with pure fruit spread and soya cream
- Fresh Fruit Salad*
- Swedish Glace soya ice cream
- Grilled nectarines sprinkled with a little brown sugar and crushed almonds
- Stewed apples and blackberries with soya custard
- Fresh fruit

SWEET SNACKS

- Fresh fruit
- Organic dried fruit
- Soya yogurt
- Sesame seed bar
- Fruit strips
- Gluten-/dairy-free scone with pure fruit spread

SAVOURY SNACKS

- Rice cakes/corn cakes with pure fruit spread/nut butter
- Small amount of unsalted nuts and seeds
- Flavoured rice cakes
- Kettle crisps
- Mini poppadums

WEEK 4 SUGGESTED MENUS

DAY 1

BREAKFAST

Soya yogurt with chopped almonds, pine nuts, a few raisins and a slice of chopped melon

LUNCH

Chicken drumstick with Beetroot and Cabbage Salad*

DINNER

Japanese Sardines* with rice and Watercress, Fennel and Lemon Salad*

DESSERT

Gooseberry Jelly*

DAY 2

BREAKFAST
Corn flakes with a few chopped pecan nuts, a chopped banana and soya milk

LUNCH
Orange and Carrot Soup* with Cornbread* and Root Salad*

DINNER
Lamb and Apricot Pilaff* with braised artichoke hearts, green beans and carrots

DESSERT
Cranberry Sorbet*

DAY 3

BREAKFAST
Wake Up Yogurt Shake* blended with 2 tbsp Wake Up Sprinkle*

LUNCH
Mushroom omelette with Beansprout Salad*

DINNER
Nut and Vegetable Loaf* with braised fennel, celery and mangetout

DESSERT
Peach Sundae*

DAY 4

BREAKFAST
Wake Up Muesli* with chopped fresh fruit and soya yogurt

LUNCH
Vegetarian pâté and crudités with corn chips

DINNER
Steak with jacket potato, baked onions and Green Salad*

DESSERT
Fresh Fruit Salad*

DAY 5

BREAKFAST
Poached cod with grilled mushrooms and tomatoes

LUNCH
Bean and Carrot Soup* with Summer Salad*

DINNER
Haddock Kedgeree*

DESSERT
Rhubarb and Ginger Mousse*

DAY 6

BREAKFAST
Wake Up Muesli* with chopped fresh fruit and soya yogurt

LUNCH
Jacket potato with tuna filling, and Ginger and Carrot Salad*

DINNER
Mexican Stuffed Eggs* with sweetcorn, French beans and braised fennel

DESSERT
Apple Custard*

DAY 7

BREAKFAST
Scrambled eggs with two rice cakes or corn crispbreads

LUNCH
Bean and Carrot Soup* with a Stuffed Pepper*

DINNER
Almond Trout* with mangetout, carrots and cauliflower

DESSERT
Dried Fruit Compote*

STAGE 1 – SAMPLE VEGETARIAN MENUS

FAST OPTIONS

DAY 1

BREAKFAST
Corn flakes, two tablespoons of golden linseeds and chopped fresh fruit with soya milk

LUNCH
Jacket potato with hummus and salad with balsamic dressing

DINNER
Mushroom and Tomato Omelette* with courgettes and mangetout

DAY 2

BREAKFAST
Wake Up Muesli* with chopped fresh fruit and soya milk

LUNCH
Bean Salad*

DINNER
Corn pasta with tomato sauce, pine kernels and fresh herbs

DAY 3

BREAKFAST
Boiled egg with rice cakes/corn crispbread or alternative soldiers

LUNCH
Puy Lentil Soup with salad

DINNER
Mixed Vegetable and Almond Stir-fry* with rice noodles

DAY 4

BREAKFAST
Soya yogurt, chopped nuts, seeds and fresh fruit

LUNCH
Beans on wheat-free toast

DINNER
Vegetarian sushi with salad

DAY 5

BREAKFAST
Fruit salad with linseeds and soya yogurt

LUNCH
Vegetarian pâté and crudités with corn chips

DINNER
Tofu and vegetable stir-fry

DAY 6

BREAKFAST
Scrambled egg, mushroom and tomatoes with wheat-free toast or crispbreads

LUNCH
Plain omelette and salad

DINNER
Corn tacos, refried beans, salsa, guacamole and salad

DAY 7

BREAKFAST
Fruit shake with soya milk, banana, berries and ground almonds

LUNCH
Polenta with Grilled Vegetables*

DINNER
Barbequed tofu and vegetable kebabs with salad

REGULAR OPTIONS

DAY 1

BREAKFAST
Wake Up Muesli* with chopped fresh fruit and soya milk

LUNCH
Bean Salad

DINNER
Quorn and vegetable kebabs served with brown rice, sweet-corn and mangetout

DESSERT
Fruit Snow*

DAY 2

BREAKFAST
Two slices of alternative toast with organic nut butter

LUNCH
Home-made or 'homestyle' fresh soup

DINNER
Vegetable and tofu curry with rice and spinach

DESSERT
Fresh Fruit Salad*

DAY 3

BREAKFAST
Soya yogurt with chopped almonds, pine nuts, a few raisins and a slice of chopped melon

LUNCH
Hummus, crudités, corn chips and a large salad

DINNER
Spinach and mushroom omelette with broccoli, carrots and new potatoes

DESSERT
Stewed apple and blackberries with home-made soya custard or soya yogurt

---

DAY 4

BREAKFAST
Wake Up Yogurt Shake* with 2 tbsp of Wake Up Sprinkle* blended in

LUNCH
Jacket potato with baked beans and a side salad

DINNER
Corn spaghetti with a tomato and basil sauce with a few toasted pine nuts

DESSERT

Meringue with fresh strawberries and a little soya cream

DAY 5

BREAKFAST

Corn flakes with almonds and sultanas with soya milk

LUNCH

Scrambled or poached eggs on alternative toast

DINNER

Mixed beans in tomato sauce served with spinach, sweetcorn and brown rice

DESSERT

Soya yogurt with a few sunflower seeds and a chopped pear

DAY 6

BREAKFAST

Boiled egg with grilled tomatoes and mushrooms and two alternative crackers or alternative soldiers

LUNCH

Grilled Mediterranean vegetables (peppers, courgettes, red onions, aubergine and garlic), marinated in balsamic vinegar, olive oil and lemon juice

DINNER

Gluten-/dairy-free veggie sausages with new potatoes, broccoli, cauliflower and carrots

DESSERT

Dried Fruit Compote*

DAY 7

BREAKFAST

Gluten-free pancakes with Dried Fruit Compote* filling and soya yogurt

LUNCH

Jacket potato with hummus, chopped avocado and a large salad

DINNER

Quorn or tofu stir-fry with vegetables, and brown rice or rice noodles

DESSERT

Swedish Glace soya ice cream with stewed berries

DAY 8

BREAKFAST

Wake Up Yogurt Shake*
Two slices gluten-free toast with pure fruit spread

LUNCH
Spinach and sweet potato omelette with salad

DINNER
Quorn chilli with brown rice and tomato salsa

DESSERT
Gluten-free scone with pure fruit spread

DAY 9

BREAKFAST
Wake Up Muesli* with soya or rice milk and fresh strawberries

LUNCH
Home-made or 'homestyle' leek and potato soup with rice cakes

DINNER
Vegetarian gluten-/dairy-free cutlet with fresh vegetables and new potatoes

DESSERT
Raspberry, mango and coconut milk soya smoothie

DAY 10

BREAKFAST
Corn flakes with Wake Up Sprinkle*, a chopped banana and soya or rice milk

LUNCH
Pear and walnut salad with walnut oil and balsamic vinegar dressing

DINNER
Gluten-/dairy-free tofu burgers with mashed potatoes and baked beans

DESSERT
Summer berries with soya yogurt and a few almonds

DAY 11

BREAKFAST
Gluten-free Pancakes* with maple syrup, a banana and chopped nuts

LUNCH
Jacket potato with hummus and a large salad

DINNER
Mushroom and herb risotto with mangetout and baby sweetcorn

DESSERT
Baked Apples* with soya cream

DAY 12

BREAKFAST
Dried Fruit Compote* with Wake Up Sprinkle* and soya yogurt

LUNCH
Stir-fried baby spinach with garlic and mushrooms served with brown rice

DINNER
Stuffed Peppers* with salad

DESSERT
Banana and Tofu Cream*

DAY 13

BREAKFAST
Mixed berry smoothie
Two slices alternative toast with Pure margarine

LUNCH
Grilled peppers, courgettes and tomatoes drizzled with balsamic vinegar, lemon juice and olive oil, served warm with salad and pine nuts

DINNER
Tomato and basil sauce with pine nuts and corn pasta

DESSERT
Grilled pineapple sprinkled with brown sugar and lemon juice

DAY 14

BREAKFAST
Scrambled eggs, mushrooms and tomatoes with rice cakes/ corn crispbread or alternative soldiers

LUNCH
Stir-fried tofu with a large salad plus Wake Up Sprinkle*

DINNER
Corn tacos with mixed spicy beans, guacamole and salsa

DESSERT
Soya yogurt with fresh fruit and a few nuts and seeds

DAY 15

BREAKFAST
Wake Up Muesli* with chopped fresh fruit and soya milk

LUNCH
Puy Lentil Soup* with Corn-bread*

DINNER
Nut and Vegetable Loaf* with Watercress, Fennel and Lemon Salad*

DESSERT
Fruit Snow*

DAY 16

BREAKFAST
Two slices of alternative toast with organic nut butter

LUNCH
Herb Tofu* with Tomato and Celery Salad*

DINNER
Vegetable Curry* with rice and spinach

DESSERT
Fresh Fruit Salad*

DAY 17

BREAKFAST
Soya yogurt with chopped almonds, pine nuts, a few raisins and a slice of chopped melon

LUNCH
Vegetarian pâté and crudités with corn crispbreads or rice cakes

DINNER
Broccoli and cauliflower in a white sauce (made with cornflour) and jacket potato

DESSERT
Gooseberry Jelly*

DAY 18

BREAKFAST
Wake Up Yogurt Shake* with 2 tbsp Wake Up Sprinkle* blended in

LUNCH
Bean Salad* with jacket potato

DINNER
Root Veggie Bake* with broccoli and courgettes

DESSERT
Apple Custard*

DAY 19

BREAKFAST
Corn flakes with chopped pecan nuts, chopped dried apricots, plus a chopped fresh banana with soya milk

LUNCH
Puy Lentil Soup* with Cauliflower and Carrot Salad*

DINNER
Bean and Tomato Hotpot* with cauliflower and jacket potato

DESSERT
Jellied Grapefruit*

DAY 20

BREAKFAST
Boiled egg with grilled tomatoes and mushrooms and two alternative crackers or alternative soldiers

LUNCH
Bean Salad* with jacket potato

DINNER
Steamed salmon with vegetables and rice

DESSERT
Banana and Tofu Cream*

DAY 21

BREAKFAST
Corn and Rice Pancakes* with Dried Fruit Compote* filling and soya yogurt

LUNCH
Beans on alternative toast with Green Salad*

DINNER
Mexican Stuffed Eggs* with rice and steamed red peppers

DESSERT
Rhubarb and Ginger Mousse*

CHAPTER 15

Real Life Diet – stage 2

Congratulations on completing Stage 1 of the Real Life Diet! By now, if you have managed to stick to the plan, you should be feeling lighter, more toned, aware of muscles you had forgotten you had, plus enjoying much more energy. If you have fallen by the wayside in the last week or so, or you would like to lose more weight before moving on to reintroduce new foods, simply repeat another two to four weeks of Stage 1, before moving on to Stage 2.

During Stage 2 we will be introducing food groups one by one, to see how your body reacts. Once you have cleared your system during Stage 1, you should find that your body will become amazingly good at helping you to identify the things it likes and dislikes. It communicates via signs and symptoms, allowing you to become a 'nutritional detective'. Very often, when the immune system is impaired, and the body reacts to certain foods or drinks, the chemicals produced may make you feel unwell in some way. The symptoms can vary from a headache, even a full-blown migraine, to eczema, nettle rash (urticaria), rhinitis, asthma, abdominal bloating and discomfort, constipation, diarrhoea, wind, anxiety, irritability, insomnia, and possibly premenstrual tension, panic attacks or even feelings of total exhaustion. The reaction may even push your weight back up, which gives you an instant clue that all is not well.

FOCUS ON WEEK 5

During this first week of Stage 2, dairy products are back on the menu, beginning with milk, followed by yogurt, then cheese and butter. You will need to introduce one variety of dairy products at a time over a period of a few days, to enable your body to report back to you. If you introduce several types of products too close together, you will only end up getting confused, and have to begin the process again.

As a general rule, you should allow five days between introducing each new food, giving the body plenty of time to respond if it is going to.

If and when you do have a reaction to individual food groups, you may feel that you have had a setback, as you may feel less well and even gain some weight. In fact, any reaction should be regarded as a positive step. It means that you have discovered some foods that don't really suit your body at the moment. A reaction, should it occur, may range from mild to severe, but is not likely to last for more than a few days, gradually wearing off. If you do experience a reaction, you will need to stop eating the suspect foods for now.

Alcohol should be introduced separately in moderate amounts, unless you know that it aggravates symptoms like headaches or thrush. I recommend no more than three units of alcohol per week at this stage, equivalent to about two glasses of wine, as apart from the fact that alcohol knocks most nutrients sideways, it is also full of calories! For your reference, one unit equals one glass of wine, or half a pint of beer or lager, one spirit or one sherry or vermouth. Alcohol is not included in the menus for Stage 2; rather I have left it up to you. Do keep careful notes when you begin introducing alcohol as repeated reports show that it does decrease well-being in large numbers of individuals.

Don't forget to carry on filling in your diary each day. It becomes an even more important record during Stage 2, as from it you will be able to track any possible reactions to food or drink. It is also important to list your personal reasons for wanting to be slimmer and feel healthier. Research shows that people who list the consequences of dieting, both positive and negative, and remind themselves of it regularly do twice as well on their diets as people who don't. Remember also to refer to the list of the positive and negative consequences of following the healthy eating plan that you made previously; you can carry this around and refer to it prior to eating or exercising.

Eat your main meals from a small plate: a well-stocked medium-sized lunch or breakfast plate looks more satisfying than a large dinner plate only half filled.

Remember. . .

- Leave five days between reintroducing new foods

- Keep alcohol to no more than three units a week

- Fill in your diary every day

- Eat from a small plate

Now it's time to look at what you can eat during this week.
(* = see recipe in Chapter 17)

BREAKFASTS

- Corn flakes with chopped fruit and nuts and semi-skimmed milk
- Wake Up Muesli* with natural bio yogurt and semi-skimmed milk
- Wake Up Yogurt Shake* with 2 tbsp of Wake Up Sprinkle* blended in

- Rice flakes soaked overnight in semi-skimmed milk served with Dried Fruit Compote*
- Gluten-free bread toasted with scrambled eggs and grilled mushrooms
- Natural bio yogurt with fresh fruit and unsalted nuts and seeds
- Cornflakes with semi-skimmed milk, a handful of raisins and a few sunflower seeds

LUNCHES

- Cheese and spinach omelette with salad
- Greek Salad*
- Home-made or 'homestyle' soup
- Cheese salad, eg Edam, Cheddar, cottage cheese
- Falafel with hummus and salad
- Jacket potato with cottage cheese and salad
- Tinned mackerel in tomato sauce with baby spinach and water-cress salad
- Rice cakes with cottage cheese or Edam and salad
- Goats' cheese grilled with cherry tomatoes and courgettes served with salad
- Mozzarella, basil and tomato salad with an olive oil and balsamic vinegar dressing

DINNERS

- Hard-boiled egg and grated cheese salad
- Lamb steak, oven chips and salad
- Oven-roasted Mediterranean vegetables with feta cheese
- Fresh grilled mackerel marinated in lemon juice and black pepper served with brown rice and salad
- Vegetable stir-fry with halloumi cheese
- Poached cod in a white sauce with steamed broccoli, spinach and new potatoes

- Spanish omelette with goats' cheese and potato wedges
- Chicken breast marinated in yogurt and spices served with a jacket potato
- Cauliflower and broccoli cheese

DESSERTS

- Blackberries with Hazelnut Cheese*
- Rice pudding with mixed berries
- Natural bio yogurt with stewed fruit
- Stewed rhubarb with custard
- Soaked brown rice flakes in semi-skimmed milk with ground cinnamon and ginger
- Frozen yogurt

SNACKS

- Bio yogurt
- Small amounts of low-fat cheese with rice cakes or alternative toast
- Fresh fruit
- Unsalted nuts and seeds
- Small piece of cheese with an apple
- Cottage cheese, fresh pineapple and a few sunflower seeds

WEEK 5 SUGGESTED MENUS

DAY 1

BREAKFAST
Wake Up Yogurt Shake* with two rice cakes and peanut butter

LUNCH
Jacket potato with hummus and salad

DINNER
Lamb steak, oven chips and salad

DESSERT
Natural bio yogurt with stewed fruit

DAY 2

BREAKFAST
Natural bio yogurt with fresh fruit and unsalted nuts and seeds

LUNCH
Home-made or 'homestyle' soup with alternative bread

DINNER
Poached cod with herbs and steamed broccoli, spinach and new potatoes

DESSERT
Fresh Fruit Salad* with bio yogurt and a few almonds and sunflower seeds

---

DAY 3

BREAKFAST
Corn flakes with semi-skimmed milk, a handful of raisins and a few sunflower seeds

LUNCH
Falafel with hummus, guacamole, tomato salsa and salad

DINNER
Chicken breast marinated in yogurt and spices served with a jacket potato

DESSERT
Stewed rhubarb and cinnamon with custard

DAY 4

BREAKFAST
Wake Up Muesli* with natural bio yogurt and semi-skimmed milk

LUNCH
Cheese and spinach omelette with salad

DINNER
Vegetable stir-fry with halloumi cheese

DESSERT
Banana and raspberry smoothie made with semi-skimmed milk and bio yogurt

---

DAY 5

BREAKFAST
Scrambled eggs on alternative toast with a little butter

LUNCH
Goats' cheese grilled with cherry tomatoes served with salad

DINNER
Fresh grilled mackerel marinated in lemon juice and black pepper served with brown rice and salad

DESSERT
Blackberries with Hazelnut Cheese*

DAY 6

BREAKFAST
Wake Up Muesli* with natural bio yogurt and semi-skimmed milk

LUNCH
Jacket potato with cold turkey and a large salad

DINNER
Cauliflower and broccoli cheese

DESSERT
Frozen yogurt

DAY 7

BREAKFAST
Mushroom and cheese omelette on alternative toast with a little butter

LUNCH
Falafel with hummus and salad and a few rice cakes

DINNER
Oven-roasted Mediterranean vegetables with chicken and feta cheese

DESSERT
Rice pudding with summer berries

FOCUS ON WEEK 6

Week 5 should have revealed whether dairy products suit your system right now. If you had no adverse reactions to any of the dairy products you can continue to include them in your menu. If you are unsure, look over your diaries to check to see how you felt on the individual dairy foods and drinks. In order to maintain your feeling of well-being it is better only to continue with those foods that made you feel well. If you did develop any symptoms, including diarrhoea, catarrh, skin irritation, weight gain or a loss of energy, you should ideally continue to exclude these foods, and try them again during the Stage 2 Review.

During the coming week you will be introducing the whole grains oats and rye, and the same rules apply as with reintroducing dairy.

Introduce each food gradually, keeping notes, and weighing yourself at least every few days to see whether you gain any of the lost pounds. There are a variety of foods to try. The oat-based foods include oatcakes, porridge oats, oat crunchy cereals and oat milk, and the rye foods consist of rye crackers, such as Ryvita (look at the labels though, as some contain wheat flour), pure rye bread (The Village Bakery make a good rye bread), pumpernickel and rye flour.

Start with one of the grains only, either oats or rye, and don't move on to the next grain until you have decided whether your body wants to continue with the first grain with which you have just experimented. If you get a positive reaction you can continue to include this grain in your menu, and if not leave it to one side until you reach the Stage 2 Review.

These grains can sometimes produce gut symptoms, ranging from indigestion to bloating and constipation. They can also affect your mood, make you feel anxious and cause a downturn in energy levels, as well as causing weight gain if they produce an antibody reaction within the body. Keep careful diaries and watch out for these symptoms. You may be fine with both types of whole grain, only one type, or neither. It is simply a question of 'suck it and see'.

It is important not to change any other aspect of your diet and lifestyle while you are trying these new foods, for if you do experience a reaction you need to know for certain that there was no other possible cause.

By now you should have got the hang of reading your body's messages. You have done well to have got this far and deserve a pat on the back. Why not treat yourself to a new outfit to show off your new shape?

Remember. . .

- You should by now be noticing the difference those lost pounds make. Your clothes should feel looser and your body should be beginning to feel toned.

- Review your long-term goals and write down your targets. Ensure your targets are realistic and span an adequate amount of time, bearing in mind that weight loss on any healthy eating plan tends to slow down as time goes on.

- Make your main mealtime sacred so that you can really enjoy your food. Eat with your family or friends instead of eating in front of the television, and relax as you eat, chewing your food slowly, while enjoying the flavours.

Now it's time to look at what you can eat during this week. (* = see recipe in Chapter 17)

BREAKFASTS

- Oat crunchy cereal with chopped fruit and nuts with low-fat yogurt
- Porridge made with semi-skimmed milk served with stewed fruit
- Wake Up Muesli* with a chopped banana, with semi-skimmed milk
- Banana and mango fruit smoothie made with semi-skimmed milk and natural bio yogurt
- Wake Up Yogurt Shake*, plus two Ryvita with pure fruit spread
- 100% pure rye bread toasted with two poached or boiled eggs
- Oatcakes or Ryvita with pure fruit spread or nut (almond, cashew, peanut) butter
- Two-egg mushroom omelette with 100% pure rye bread

LUNCHES

- Rye bread sandwiches with fish, poultry, cheese or egg filling
- Home-made or 'homestyle' soup with rye bread or oatcakes
- Jacket potato with hummus and salad
- Sardines in olive oil with a salad and oatcakes
- Scrambled eggs on 100% rye bread toast
- Natural bio yogurt with chopped fresh fruit and nuts and seeds
- Oven-roasted Mediterranean vegetables with feta cheese
- Spinach and sweet potato omelette served with salad
- Falafel with hummus on open rye bread sandwiches
- Ryvita with cottage cheese, fresh pineapple and a few sunflower seeds

DINNERS

- Tuna steak marinated in lemon juice, garlic and black pepper, then grilled and served with broccoli, mangetout and new potatoes
- Stir-fry chicken or prawns and vegetables served with brown rice or rice noodles
- Pilchards in tomato sauce with salad and a jacket potato
- Oaty Vegetable Crumble*
- Chicken breast brushed with pesto, grilled and served with fresh vegetables
- Broccoli and cauliflower cheese
- Lamb Kebabs*
- Ratatouille with brown rice and a little grated cheese
- Salmon and broccoli quiche (pastry made with rye flour) with salad
- Roasted veggie quiche (pastry made with rye flour) with salad

DESSERTS

- Tropical Crumble*
- Oats soaked in semi-skimmed milk, served with bio yogurt, stewed apple and a little pure maple syrup
- Rye pancakes with fresh fruit and bio yogurt
- Grilled fresh pineapple sprinkled with a little brown sugar, cinnamon and lemon juice, served with natural bio yogurt
- Bio yogurt with chopped fresh fruit and Wake Up Sprinkle*
- Fresh Fruit Salad* with yogurt

SNACKS

- Rye bread with a little portion of cheese
- Oatcakes with nut butter or honey
- Crunchy oat cereal bar
- Fresh fruit
- Bio yogurt
- Handful of unsalted nuts and seeds
- Dried fruit

WEEK 6 SUGGESTED MENUS

DAY 1

BREAKFAST
Oat crunchy cereal with chopped fruit and nuts with semi-skimmed milk or soya milk

LUNCH
Jacket potato with hummus and salad

DINNER
Tuna steak marinated in lemon juice, garlic and black pepper, than grilled and served with broccoli, mangetout and new potatoes

DESSERT
Grilled fresh pineapple sprinkled with a little brown sugar, cinnamon and lemon juice served with natural bio yogurt

---

DAY 2

BREAKFAST
Wake Up Muesli* with a chopped banana, with semi-skimmed milk

LUNCH
Sardines in olive oil with a salad and oatcakes

DINNER
Chicken breast brushed with pesto sauce, grilled and served with fresh vegetables

DESSERT
Bio yogurt with chopped fresh fruit and Wake Up Sprinkle*

DAY 3

BREAKFAST
Banana and mango fruit smoothie made with semi-skimmed milk or soya milk
Two oatcakes with pure fruit spread

LUNCH
Oven-roasted vegetables with feta cheese

DINNER
Oaty Vegetable Crumble*

DESSERT
Fresh Fruit Salad* with yoghurt and nuts and seeds

DAY 4

BREAKFAST

Porridge made with semi-skimmed milk served with stewed fruit

LUNCH

Spinach and sweet potato omelette served with salad

DINNER

Stir-fry chicken or prawns and vegetables served with brown rice or rice noodles

DESSERT

Tropical Crumble*

(NB If you didn't feel so well on oats, wait a few days before trying rye and replace the oats on days 4 to 7 with rice and corn products.)

DAY 5

BREAKFAST

Corn flakes with a chopped banana and a few nuts and seeds

LUNCH

Falafel with hummus on open rye-bread sandwiches

DINNER

Broccoli and cauliflower cheese

DESSERT

Rice pudding served with puréed summer berries

DAY 6

BREAKFAST

Wake Up Yogurt Shake*, plus two Ryvita with pure fruit spread

LUNCH

Rye-bread sandwiches with fish, poultry, cheese or egg filling served with a salad

DINNER

Lamb Kebabs* with assorted fresh vegetables and new potatoes

DESSERT

Banana with home-made vanilla custard

DAY 7

BREAKFAST

Two-egg mushroom omelette with 100% pure rye bread

LUNCH

Home-made vegetable soup with oatcakes or Ryvita

DINNER

Pilchards in tomato sauce with salad and a jacket potato

DESSERT

Rye pancakes with fresh fruit or stewed fruit compote, served with natural bio yogurt

FOCUS ON WEEK 7

If you have introduced both oats and rye successfully, without any symptoms or adverse effects, you can now move on to introducing foods containing white flour. If, however, you have gained some weight or some of your old symptoms have returned to greet you, you should go back on to the basic diet, but including dairy products, if you were fine with those, for another week or two until things settle down.

I have had many clients who have been so happy on Stage 1 of the Real Life Diet, and so pleased to be feeling good while at the same time losing weight, that they were reluctant to make any changes. So, if you don't yet feel happy about appearing in public in your shorts or in the bikini of your choice, or you simply felt better on the basic diet, feel free to continue for as long as you like, for unlike most ordinary weight-loss diets, this is an eating plan that is nutritionally balanced for the long term.

Those of you who are going on to introduce foods containing white flour may be surprised to find that the introduction of white flour comes before wholemeal products, which are perceived to be better for us. Sound reasoning is involved here. Whole-grain products, including bran, have much higher gluten content than refined white flour, and are therefore more likely to cause a reaction. So it is always best to start introducing foods made with white flour, such as bread, pasta, pastry, pizza and sauces, to test the waters, remembering to combine them with other foods in order to lower their GI score.

The best thing to try first is French bread, made with French flour, which is now widely available, for French flour has far lower gluten content than British-grown wheat. That means you can start tucking into baguettes, which you have probably been dreaming of for the last six weeks. Make sure you keep careful notes in your diary during this process, and weigh yourself regularly, watching out for weight surges, flagging energy levels or bowel symptoms such as bloating, wind, constipation or diarrhoea. You will see from this week's menu that we advise the introduction of small quantities of bread initially, gradually increasing the number of servings and portion sizes as the week progresses.

Remember. . .

- You may begin to notice that certain foods seem to make you feel bloated or result in a rapid drop in energy levels or even bring on a headache. Keep an eye on how you feel after eating and note down the symptoms you are experiencing in your diary. After a few weeks, you may well see a pattern emerging, which will make it easier to spot the suspect foods.

- Give yourself a pat on the back at this stage, but make a point of not getting complacent. Consider the changes you have had to make to get to this point, and think twice before returning to your old habits.

- Review your goals at this point and continue with the plan for as long as you feel it is appropriate.

Now it's time to look at what you can eat during this week.
(* = see recipe in Chapter 17)

BREAKFASTS

- Wake Up Muesli* with chopped fresh fruit and semi-skimmed milk
- Scrambled eggs with a toasted bagel
- Bio yogurt with chopped fresh fruit and Wake Up Sprinkle*
- Two boiled eggs with white toasted soldiers
- Corn flakes with chopped unsalted nuts and seeds with semi-skimmed milk
- Porridge made with semi-skimmed milk with stewed apple, cinnamon and ginger
- Ryvita with nut butter and a banana

- Pancakes with stewed apple, sultanas and cinnamon and bio yogurt
- Two slices of white toast with pure fruit spread or a little honey

LUNCHES

- Baked beans on toast
- Hummus and falafel with a mixed salad and pitta bread
- Jacket potato with baked beans
- Spinach and mushroom quiche served with salad
- Oven-roasted vegetables and hummus served with ciabatta bread
- Tuna and pasta salad
- Cheese salad with French bread
- Tuna and mozzarella toasted sandwich
- Greek Salad* with pitta bread
- French bread pizza topped with tomatoes, basil, mozzarella, olives and prawns

DINNERS

- Fish in breadcrumbs with spinach, broccoli and new potatoes
- Grilled chicken breast marinated in lemon, garlic and black pepper with assorted fresh vegetables
- Flour tortillas with mince or beans, guacamole and salsa
- Spaghetti bolognaise
- Pasta with tomato and basil sauce with spinach, mushrooms and pine kernels
- Home-made Pizza Base* with topping of your choice
- Poached salmon with assorted fresh vegetables
- Mushroom quiche with a large salad and potato wedges
- Tomato and basil sauce with tagliatelle, sprinkled with a little grated Parmesan cheese
- Cherry tomatoes, mozzarella and basil marinated in olive oil and balsamic vinegar served with fresh pasta

DESSERTS

- Apple Charlotte*
- Pancakes with stewed fruit and natural bio yogurt
- Summer berry crumble served with natural bio yogurt
- Fresh Fruit Salad* with toasted almonds and pumpkin seeds
- Summer pudding
- Stewed prunes and apricots served with natural yogurt
- Rice pudding served with raspberry purée and a few flaked almonds
- Banana custard with a few chopped nuts

WEEK 7 SUGGESTED MENUS

DAY 1

BREAKFAST
Bio yogurt with chopped fresh fruit and Wake Up Sprinkle*

LUNCH
Jacket potato with baked beans

DINNER
Pasta with tomato and basil sauce with spinach, mushrooms and pine kernels

DESSERT
Apple Charlotte*

DAY 2

BREAKFAST
Scrambled eggs with a toasted bagel

LUNCH
Tuna and mozzarella toasted sandwich

DINNER

Grilled chicken breast marinated in lemon, garlic and black pepper with assorted fresh vegetables

DESSERT

Summer berry crumble served with natural bio yogurt

DAY 3

BREAKFAST

Two boiled eggs with white toasted soldiers

LUNCH

Spinach and mushroom quiche served with salad

DINNER

Poached salmon with assorted fresh vegetables

DESSERT

Fresh Fruit Salad* with toasted almonds and pumpkin seeds

DAY 4

BREAKFAST

Pancakes with stewed apple, sultanas and cinnamon and bio yogurt

LUNCH

Hummus and falafel with a mixed salad

DINNER

Home-made Pizza Base* with topping of your choice

DESSERT

Rice pudding served with raspberry purée and a few flaked almonds

DAY 5

BREAKFAST
Wake Up Muesli* with chopped fresh fruit and semi-skimmed milk

LUNCH
Jacket potato with cottage cheese, sweetcorn and a large salad

DINNER
Spaghetti bolognaise or tomato and basil sauce with tagliatelle, sprinkled with a little grated Parmesan cheese

DESSERT
Stewed prunes and apricots served with natural yogurt

DAY 6

BREAKFAST
Ryvita or two slices of white toast with nut butter and a mashed banana

LUNCH
Oven-roasted vegetables and hummus served with ciabatta bread

DINNER
Pasta with tomato and basil sauce with spinach, mushrooms and pine kernels

DESSERT
Banana custard with a few chopped nuts

DAY 7

BREAKFAST
Corn flakes with chopped unsalted nuts and seeds with semi-skimmed milk

LUNCH
Greek Salad* with pitta bread

DINNER

Jacket potato with tinned mackerel in tomato sauce, served with a large salad

DESSERT

Summer pudding with home-made custard or natural yogurt

FOCUS ON WEEK 8

As weight loss has been your main motivation for following the Real Life Diet, be wary about introducing whole-wheat products before you have reached your target weight. In my experience, many people who are not in brilliant nutritional shape, and whose immune system may not be operating in an optimum fashion, may retain fluid as part of an adverse chemical reaction to whole wheat or bran, or display bowel symptoms or fatigue.

Once you are feeling well and have lost the desired weight, feel free to reintroduce whole-wheat products gradually over a period of a week or two, all the while keeping careful notes of any symptoms that may occur and keeping an eye on your weight. If the scales show that the pounds are creeping back on – beware. It may be that at this point you can tolerate whole wheat in small quantities, meaning that you can eat it 'socially' rather than as part of your everyday diet.

If your reaction to whole wheat is severe, it is best to exclude it completely from your diet for at least the next few months, before having another attempt at its reintroduction. You will have discovered by now that there are plenty of delicious alternatives freely available, and it may even be that you are quite happy with your current diet, and stopped pining for whole wheat some time ago.

If you decide that wheat, or whole wheat, are no-go areas at the moment, you simply need to go back on to the basic diet for the next week or two in order the drop the pounds you gained while doing the experiment. You may be surprised by the rapid loss of weight once off wheat again, but this may be due to loss of fluid collected to dilute the chemical reaction in your body to the wheat.

By the end of this week you will essentially have completed Stage 2 of the Real Life Diet, and it will be time to look at Stage 3 – your plan for the longer term.

Remember. . .

- Eat regular meals three times each day with one or two between-meal snacks. It is better to eat four or five small meals each day, than guzzle large meals because you are so hungry.

- Women, in the week before their period, should bear in mind that their calorie requirements rise by approximately 500 calories per day.

- Making time for yourself is probably one of the most important long-term resolutions you should be considering. If you lead a hectic life write your exercise and relaxation time into your diary like any business appointment. That way you stand a good chance of preserving that special time for yourself.

Now it's time to look at what you can eat during this week. (* = see recipe in Chapter 17)

BREAKFASTS

- Wholemeal toast with nut butter or pure fruit spread
- Wake Up Muesli* with semi-skimmed milk and natural bio yogurt
- Scrambled eggs on wholemeal toast

- Corn flakes with chopped pecan nuts, fresh pear and semi-skimmed milk
- Natural bio yogurt with Wake Up Sprinkle*
- Stewed prunes with natural bio yogurt and crunchy oat cereal
- Pancakes made with wholemeal flour, served with stewed apple, sultanas and cinnamon
- Wholemeal muffin with a poached egg, and mushrooms and tomatoes lightly sautéed in olive oil

LUNCHES

- Pilchards in tomato sauce with salad and wholemeal bread
- Jacket potato with hummus and a large salad
- Scrambled eggs and baked beans on wholemeal toast
- Chicken, avocado and tomato wholemeal sandwich
- Omelette with a large salad
- Wholemeal mushroom quiche with salad
- Cherry tomato, basil and mozzarella salad with wholemeal pitta bread
- 'Homestyle' vegetable soup with a chunk of wholemeal bread

DINNERS

- Grilled plaice with fresh vegetables and brown rice
- Turkey and green pepper kebabs with hummus, salad and wholemeal pitta bread
- Stir-fry vegetables and chicken with brown rice or egg noodles
- Wholemeal pizza with spinach and goats' cheese served with salad
- Poached salmon with assorted fresh vegetables
- Ratatouille with wholemeal pasta and a salad with olive oil and balsamic vinegar
- Oven-roasted Mediterranean vegetables with mozzarella cheese
- Wholemeal salmon and broccoli quiche with salad
- Wholemeal pasta with a tomato and herb sauce
- Cold chicken with a jacket potato and large salad

DESSERTS

- Wholemeal apple and cinnamon crumble with home-made custard or natural yogurt
- Wholemeal pancakes with stewed summer berries and Greek yogurt
- Fresh Fruit Salad* with yogurt and a few nuts and seeds
- Wholemeal date slice with natural bio yogurt
- Natural bio yogurt with honey and a banana
- Wholemeal bread and butter pudding with home-made custard
- Grilled pineapple marinated in lemon juice, and a little brown sugar, served with toasted pecans and fromage frais

WEEK 8 SUGGESTED MENUS

DAY 1

BREAKFAST
Wholemeal toast with nut butter or pure fruit spread

LUNCH
Jacket potato with hummus and a large salad

DINNER
Grilled plaice with fresh vegetables and brown rice

DESSERT
Wholemeal bread and butter pudding with home-made custard

DAY 2

BREAKFAST
Wake Up Muesli* with semi-skimmed milk and natural bio yogurt

LUNCH
Wholemeal mushroom quiche with salad

DINNER

Stir-fry vegetables and chicken with brown rice or egg noodles

DESSERT

Grilled pineapple marinated in lemon juice, and sugar, served with toasted pecans and Greek yogurt

---

DAY 3

BREAKFAST

Wholemeal muffin with a poached egg, mushrooms and tomatoes lightly sautéed in olive oil

LUNCH

Home-made vegetable soup with a chunk of wholemeal bread

DINNER

Poached salmon with assorted fresh vegetables

DESSERT

Natural yogurt with honey and a banana

DAY 4

BREAKFAST

Pancakes made with wholemeal flour, served with stewed apple, sultanas and cinnamon

LUNCH

Oven-roasted Mediterranean vegetables with mozzarella cheese

DINNER

Turkey and apricot kebabs with hummus, salad and wholemeal pitta bread

DESSERT

Wholemeal date slice with natural yogurt

DAY 5

BREAKFAST
Stewed prunes with natural bio yogurt and crunchy oat cereal

LUNCH
Chicken, avocado and tomato wholemeal sandwich

DINNER
Wholemeal salmon and broccoli quiche with salad

DESSERT
Fresh Fruit Salad* with yogurt and a few nuts and seeds

DAY 6

BREAKFAST
Corn flakes with chopped pecan nuts, fresh pear with milk or soya milk

LUNCH
Mushroom omelette with a large salad

DINNER
Wholemeal pizza with spinach and goats' cheese served with salad

DESSERT
Wholemeal pancakes with stewed summer berries and Greek yogurt

---

DAY 7

BREAKFAST
Scrambled eggs on wholemeal toast

LUNCH
Jacket potato with pilchards in tomato sauce with a large salad

DINNER

Ratatouille with wholemeal pasta and a salad with olive oil, lemon juice and balsamic vinegar

DESSERT

Wholemeal apple and cinnamon crumble with home-made custard or natural yogurt

CHAPTER 16

Real Life Diet grand review – stage 3

During the next four weeks you will need to follow the plan that you have by now devised for yourself, avoiding any foods or drinks that affected either your physical or mental well-being. Continue keeping your daily diary so that you can check to ensure that you have got it right and remain symptom free without gaining any of the weight you have lost. If you are unsure about any aspect of the diet, leave out the foods or drinks that have a question mark over them for five days and then reintroduce them if you want to. Sometimes, certain foods and drinks cause undesired effects and you may decide it is best to avoid them in the long term. There is no harm in having another go at reintroducing the suspect foods or drinks a few months down the line.

By the time you reach the end of Stage 3 of the Real Life Diet you should be looking good, feeling well and aware of a better balance in your life. It will have been three months since you began the Real Life Diet and so it is time to take the tests again (see page 309), so that you can arrive at your 'after' score. So do that now. When all the scores have been entered you can then deduct the new scores from the old scores and arrive at your Personal Balance Score – this is a measure of how much progress you have made as a result of following the Real Life Diet. I would love to hear how you did and invite you to go to www.reallifeplan.com and enter your details. There is a monthly prize for the best achievement and you can swap stories with others who have also been following the Real Life Diet.

The general consensus is that the voyage through this plan is a trip through previously unknown territory. Now that you know how to interpret your body's messages and have become familiar with what it likes and dislikes, you will no doubt agree that it was worth the effort. It's amazing how much better we feel and how our relationships thrive when we are in good shape physically. A little knowledge in this case goes an awfully long way; you may feel it's only a pity that the information wasn't available to you earlier in your life.

In order to make the most of your voyage of discovery you will now need to make a plan for the longer term.

Real Life Extension Plan

You will probably be only too aware of any reactions experienced during the three stages of the Real Life Diet, but it is still worth setting a little time aside now, both to review your progress and make a plan for the future (see page 312).

- As you look through your weekly charts make a list of any foods or drinks that definitely seemed to cause a reaction, which will be known as your black list, together with another list of items that you are currently unsure of, your grey list.

- You will need to concentrate on all the products on your white list (the foods and drinks you seemed to thrive on) for the next few weeks, taking care to omit items from both the grey and black lists from your diet.

- When you feel the time is right, for example, when you are feeling really well, or when you have reached and maintained your target weight for a few months, re-test the grey list by introducing the foods back into your diet one by one, as before, leaving five days between each food.

- Another few months down the line, re-test the remaining foods on the grey list gradually, one by one as before. Sometimes when the body is in better nutritional shape your tolerance to certain foods and drinks improves.

- The foods and drinks that remain on both the grey list and the black list may be tested again several months down the line, but always individually, leaving plenty of time for any reaction to rear its head.

What about foods that seem to cause weight gain in the long term?

Once you are in better nutritional shape, it is not uncommon to be able to reintroduce foods that previously caused weight gain without any movement on the dial of your scales. However, some people continue to have an antibody reaction, and they will therefore need to be wary about introducing suspect foods (notably whole wheat) in the longer term. Wheat and bran are the two most common triggers of the classic chemical reaction with fluid retention.

To continue losing weight

If you had a considerable amount of weight to lose, and have not achieved your target weight by the end of the Real Life Diet, there is nothing to stop you continuing on the Diet for as many months as you wish. Unlike other weight loss diets you may have followed the Real Life Diet is designed to provide you with all the important nutrients your body needs to thrive in the long term and can be continued for as long as you like.

Once you have completed your weight-loss programme

There is no need to revert to your old ways of eating when you have completed the Real Life Diet. It will be much better for your health and well-being in the long term if you remain on the regime, perhaps increasing the portion sizes a little, or adding in some of the little treats listed in the dessert sections for the long term, for example. There is no harm in deviating from your basic diet on special occasions or while on holiday, as you are now armed with the knowledge of what your body really needs on a regular basis. I firmly believe that when you are well, 'a little of what you fancy does you good'.

Supplements for the long term

While I am not recommending long-term pill popping, there are times when supplements will improve the quality of life, especially when taken in gradually reducing doses. Look back at Chapter 3, where different supplements for different life stages were discussed. Everyone is different, so your long-term supplement programme, should you decide that supplements are necessary, will be the result of trial and error over the months, until you find the regime that seems to suit you. There will be times when you need to review your supplements, for example when you are actively planning to conceive, are pregnant or breastfeeding, or moving from childbearing years into the menopause. For more on this subject, see *The Natural Health Bible* (details in Recommended reading and further information on page 322).

Keep fit and make time for yourself

Unfortunately, most of us have to work at remaining in good physical and mental shape. While it may take a while and some in-depth personal persuasion to get a regular exercise programme established, it certainly gives you a regular infusion of that 'feel good factor'. So don't get complacent at the end of the Real Life Diet and think you feel so well there is no need to continue. Many have made that mistake before and lived to regret it! Enjoy your exercise time, and make time to relax on a regular basis, even if it is only for fifteen minutes per day. We all need time to reflect on our lives, on decisions that need to be made, or indeed on our achievements. The time you invest in exercise and relaxation will be repaid to you in terms of increased energy and improved mood. When you feel positive, happy and energetic you are bound to achieve more in life and, as an added bonus, to attract more interesting company.

Having helped thousands of people to help themselves to better health over the last 14 years, I really believe that in the final analysis it is up to individuals to invest in themselves. Once armed with the knowledge, which of course you now are, the quality of your health in the long term is very much in your own hands. You may regard this as a somewhat daunting prospect, but it very definitely puts you in the driving seat, and the only side-effects you are likely to experience are that you will be looking good and feeling fine for a long time to come.

CHAPTER 17

Real Life Diet Recipes

BREAKFAST – STAGES 1 and 2

Corn and Rice Pancakes

(Serves 4)

50 g (2 oz) rice flour
50 g (2 oz) cornflour
1 small egg
300 ml (10 fl oz) soya/rice milk, or skimmed at Stages 2 and 3
a little oil

1. Make a thin batter with the flours, egg and milk.
2. Use kitchen paper to wipe a small non-stick frying pan with a little oil and heat until the oil is smoking.
3. Pour a generous 2 tablespoons of batter into the pan and swirl it around to cover the base. Cook for 60 seconds.
4. Flip the pancake over and cook for a further few seconds. Set aside.
5. Repeat the procedure until you have used up all the batter.

Gluten-free Muesli

(Makes 10–12 servings)
2 mugs brown rice flakes
1 mug buckwheat flakes
½ mug sunflower seeds
½ mug chopped almonds
½ mug pumpkin seeds
⅔ mug organic raisins (optional)

1. Mix the ingredients together and store in a sealed container.
2. Serve with chopped fresh fruit and the appropriate yogurt or milk.

Gluten-free Pancakes

(Serves 4)
100 g (4 oz) gluten-free flour (available from Dove's Farm)
1 small egg
300 ml (10 fl oz) soya milk
a little oil

1. Make a thin batter with the flour, egg and milk.
2. Use kitchen paper to wipe a small non-stick frying pan with a little oil and heat until the oil is smoking.
3. Pour a generous 2 tablespoons of batter into the pan and swirl it around to cover the base. Cook for 60 seconds.
4. Flip the pancake over and cook for a further few seconds. Set aside.
5. Repeat the procedure until you have used up all the batter.

Mixed Berry Bonanza

(Serves 2)
450 ml (¾ pint) soya milk
1 cup natural bio soya yogurt
1 cup frozen mixed berries (partially thawed)
1 banana
1 tbsp ground almonds

1. Blend the fruit with the soya milk and yogurt.
2. Stir in the ground almonds thoroughly and serve immediately.

Mushroom and Tomato Omelette

(Serves 1)
2 medium eggs
soya milk
50 g (2 oz) mushrooms
2 ripe tomatoes
olive oil
freshly ground black pepper

1. Crack the eggs and beat together with a little soya milk. Season with black pepper. Put to one side.
2. Lightly sauté the mushrooms and tomatoes in a large frying pan in olive oil until golden.
3. Pour the egg and milk mixture over the mushrooms and tomatoes into the frothing pan and cook for 2–3 minutes until the underside is golden and the top is bubbling.
4. Either turn the omelette in the pan to cook the top, or put under a medium hot grill until the eggs are cooked and the omelette is firm.
5. Serve alone or with sautéed potatoes or baked beans.

Wake Up Muesli

(Makes 10–12 servings)
2½ mugs puffed rice
2 mugs corn flakes
½ mug sunflower seeds
½ mug chopped almonds
⅔ mug organic raisins

1. Mix the ingredients together and store in a sealed container.
2. Serve with chopped fresh fruit and the appropriate yogurt or milk.

(NB: If you are constipated, you will need to sprinkle 1–2 tbsp of organic linseeds on to your muesli each morning for the best results!)

Wake Up Sprinkle

Three servings per week are allowed until you have reached your target weight. Use organic seeds where possible.

(Makes 18 tbsp (1 level tbsp = 1 serving))
½ mug almonds
½ mug sunflower seeds
⅓ mug pumpkin seeds
¼ mug golden linseeds

1. Grind the ingredients together in a blender to a coarse powder consistency.
2. Store in a sealed container.

Wake Up Yogurt Shake

(Makes 2 large servings)
1 large carton of natural bio or soya yogurt
3 portions fruit of your choice, skinned and cut into segments
ice cubes (optional)

1. Blend the ingredients together in a liquidiser and serve immediately.

Variation: Blend in 2 tbsp Wake Up Sprinkle

ADDITIONAL BREAKFAST RECIPES FOR STAGE 2

Oatcakes

(Makes 12 biscuits)
25 g (1 oz) margarine
2 tbsps boiling water
225 g (8 oz) medium oatmeal
pinch of salt (or potassium-rich substitute)
¼ tsp baking powder

1. Preheat the oven to 190°C/375°F/Gas mark 5.
2. Melt the margarine in the boiling water in a bowl.
3. Add the remaining ingredients and mix to form a soft dough.
4. Roll out thinly on a floured surface and cut into 12 portions.
5. Put on to a greased baking tray and bake in the preheated oven for 25 minutes or until lightly coloured. Cool on a wire rack.

Swiss Muesli

(Serves 2)
2 cups porridge oats
1 apple, peeled and grated
1 cup raisins
300 ml (½ pint) apple juice or soya milk
1 tbsp chopped almonds
1 cup natural bio yogurt
sprinkling of ground cinnamon and ginger

1. Soak the porridge oats, grated apple and raisins for at least half an hour in the apple juice or soya milk.
2. Stir in the chopped almonds and yogurt and serve with a sprinkling of ground cinnamon and ginger.

SOUPS – STAGES 1 AND 2

Bean and Carrot Soup

(Serves 4)

1 tbsp sunflower oil
450 g (1 lb) carrots, peeled and sliced
1 large potato, diced
1 medium onion, chopped
900 ml (1½ pints) water
1 tbsp tomato purée
a good pinch of ground coriander
freshly ground black pepper
1 × 415 g (15 oz) can kidney beans, drained and rinsed
chopped fresh parsley

1. Heat the oil in a saucepan, add the vegetables and cook, stirring for 5 minutes.
2. Add the water, tomato purée, coriander and pepper to taste, and bring to the boil. Lower the heat, cover and simmer for 45 minutes.
3. Stir in the kidney beans and reheat gently.
4. Pour into individual soup bowls, garnish with parsley and serve at once.

Chicken and Spinach Soup

(Serves 4)

2 chicken breasts, skinned and each chopped into 8 pieces
600 ml (1 pint) water
2 tsp (10 ml) sunflower oil
1 onion, finely chopped
150 g (5 oz) spinach, stalks removed and leaves shredded
freshly ground black pepper
600 ml (1 pint) soya milk

1. Place the chicken and water in a saucepan, bring to the boil and simmer for 45 minutes.

2. Heat the oil and gently fry the onion for 2 minutes until translucent.
3. Remove the onion with a slotted spoon and add to the chicken and liquid.
4. Add the spinach, season with black pepper to taste, and cook for a further 5 minutes.
5. Add the soya milk and heat through before serving.

Orange and Carrot Soup

This soup can also be used as a sauce for grilled or roast meats, or cold as a salad dressing.

(Serves 2 as a soup, 4 as a sauce)
300 g (10 oz) carrots, chopped
1 medium leek, thinly sliced
360 ml (12 fl oz) vegetable stock
a pinch of thyme
75–115 ml (3–4 fl oz) orange juice
freshly ground black pepper

1. Place the carrots, leek, vegetable stock and thyme into a saucepan, bring to the boil and simmer for 30 minutes.
2. Purée the mixture in a blender or food processor.
3. Return to the saucepan, add the orange juice and season with pepper. Heat through very gently.

Puy Lentil Soup

(Serves 6–8)
450 g (1 lb) Puy lentils
1 litre (1¾ pints) water
2 tbsp sunflower oil
1 large onion, peeled and finely chopped
2 garlic cloves, crushed
1.4 litres (2½ pints) vegetable stock
1 large carrot, peeled and chopped
2 sticks celery, trimmed and chopped

1 bay leaf
freshly ground black pepper

1. Place the Puy lentils and water in a pan and bring to the boil. Boil for 2 minutes, then remove from the heat and leave to stand for 2 hours, covered. Drain.
2. Heat the oil in a saucepan and lightly brown the onion. Add the garlic and mix well.
3. Stir in the drained lentils, add the stock and bring to the boil.
4. Add the carrots, celery, bay leaf and black pepper.
5. Simmer for 45–60 minutes until the lentils are tender, then remove the bay leaf.
6. Half, or all, the soup can be puréed in a blender or food processor.

Sweet Potato, Broccoli and Spinach Soup

(Serves 6–8)
oil
1 onion, finely chopped
1 large sweet potato, peeled and diced
450 ml (¾ pint) vegetable stock
1 large head of broccoli
225 g (8 oz) spinach
150 ml (¼ pint) soya milk
seasoning to taste

1. Heat the oil in a large saucepan and soften the onion without browning.
2. Add the sweet potato and coat in the juices.
3. Add the vegetable stock, bring to the boil and simmer until the sweet potato starts to soften.
4. Add the broccoli and spinach and continue cooking over a gentle heat until all the vegetables are cooked through.
5. Blend the ingredients in the pan with a hand blender until smooth or pour into a liquidiser.
6. Stir in the soya milk and season to taste. A little more soya milk can be added for a thinner consistency.

BREAD ALTERNATIVES

Cornbread

(Makes 12 squares)

175 g (6 oz) polenta
50 g (2 oz) rice flour
50 g (2 oz) potato flour
2–3 tbsp brown sugar
2 tsp baking powder (wheat free)
1 tsp salt
300 ml (½ pint) tepid milk
2 eggs, lightly beaten
50 g (2 oz) butter, melted and cooled slightly

1. Lightly grease an 18 cm (7 in) square cake tin.
2. Put the polenta, flour, sugar, baking powder and salt into a large bowl, and make a well in the middle. Pour in the milk, eggs and butter, and beat the ingredients to form a batter.
3. Pour the mixture into the cake tin and bake in a preheated oven at 200°C/400°F/Gas mark 6 25–30 minutes until golden. Leave the cornbread to cool, then cut into squares. Serve warm or cold.

Variation: For a savoury variation to serve with chilli con carne, add 250 g (8 oz) grated Cheddar cheese, and 1 cored, seeded and finely chopped green chilli to the cornbread mixture, and proceed as directed.

Potato Farls

(Makes 12)

175 g (6 oz) plain flour
1 tbsp baking powder
50 g (2 oz) butter
45 g (1½ oz) caster sugar (unbleached)
125 g (4 oz) freshly boiled and mashed potato
3 tbsp milk

1. Sift the flour and baking powder into a bowl. Rub in the butter until the mixture resembles fine breadcrumbs. Stir in the sugar and mashed potato. Add enough milk to bind to a soft but not sticky dough.
2. Turn the dough onto a floured surface and knead lightly until blended. Roll out until 1 cm (½ in) thick and cut into rectangles.
3. Place the rectangles onto a greased baking tray and bake in a pre-heated oven at 220°C/425°F/Gas mark 7 for 12–15 minutes until risen and golden. Leave to cool on a wire rack. Serve on the day of making.

Potato and Rice Bread

(Serves 12)

275 g (10 oz) potato flour
225 g (8 oz) brown rice flour
1½ packets easy-blend yeast
1 teaspoon sugar
1 tablespoon oil
½–1 teaspoon salt
300–350ml (10–12 fl oz) hand-hot water

1. Mix together the flours and easy blend yeast.
2. Add the sugar, oil and salt and mix to a thick batter with the hand-hot water.
3. Grease and flour 2 × 450 g (1 lb) loaf tins. Divide the mixture between the two tins, cover and leave to rice in a warm place for 20-30 minutes.
4. Bake the loaves in a preheated oven at 230°C/450°F/Gas mark 8 for 35–40 minutes. The bread will slightly contract from the side of the tins when it is cooked.
5. Cool for 5 minutes in the tins and then turn on to a wire rack. Slice when cold.

Rice and Cornflour Crispbread

(Makes 12 squares or 8 'Ryvita' size shapes)
100 g (4 oz) brown rice flour
50 g (2 oz) cornflour
30 ml (2 tablespoons) oil of your choice
warm water to mix

1. Pre-heat the oven to 200°C/425°F/Gas mark 7.
2. Mix the ingredients together using enough water to make a soft dough.
3. Roll the dough out thinly on a surface dusted with rice flour. Cut into oblong biscuits and place on a greased baking tray.
4. Bake for 8–10 minutes.

LUNCHES – STAGES 1 and 2

Baked Avocado with Tuna

(Serves 4)
25 g (1 oz) sunflower margarine (Pure)
50 g (2 oz) gluten-free flour (Dove's Farm)
150 ml (¼ pint) soya milk
black pepper to taste
100 g (4 oz) can tuna in olive oil, well drained and flaked
1 tbsp lemon juice
2 large ripe avocados
25 g (1 oz) Gruyère cheese, grated
lemon slices, to garnish

1. Melt the margarine in a saucepan, stir in the flour and cook for 2 minutes, stirring constantly.
2. Remove from the heat, and gradually stir in the soya milk. Bring slowly to the boil, stirring constantly, then simmer for 2 minutes, stirring until thickened. Season with pepper and remove from the heat.

3. Stir the tuna and lemon juice into the sauce.
4. Cut the avocados in half and remove the stones. Stand the avocado halves in a baking dish, using crumpled foil, if necessary, to help them stand upright.
5. Spoon the tuna mixture on to the avocados, covering all the avocado flesh. Sprinkle with grated cheese and bake in a preheated oven at 180°C (350°F/Gas mark 4) for 15–20 minutes.
6. Transfer the avocados to serving dishes, garnish with lemon slices and serve immediately.

Chickpea Dips with Crudités

(Serves 8)

2 × 415 g (15 oz) cans chickpeas, drained and rinsed
1 garlic clove, crushed
1 tbsp fresh lemon juice
25 ml (1 fl oz) olive oil
175 ml (6 fl oz) plain Greek yogurt
freshly ground black pepper
4 tsp freshly chopped parsley
2 tsp tomato purée
sprigs of parsley, strips of red pepper and pieces of sliced lemon to garnish
a selection of raw vegetables (peppers, radishes, carrots, celery, cucumber) to serve

1. Place the chickpeas in a blender or food processor and blend until smooth.
2. Add the garlic, lemon juice, olive oil and yogurt and mix well. Add pepper to taste.
3. Transfer one-third of the mixture to a small serving bowl. Divide the rest between 2 small mixing bowls.
4. Add the chopped parsley to one, stir well and transfer to a small serving bowl.
5. Add the tomato purée to the other, stir well and transfer to another small serving bowl. Adjust seasoning if necessary.

6. Garnish the parsley dip with sprigs of parsley, the tomato dip with red pepper and the plain dip with the pieces of lemon.
7. Chop the raw vegetables into sticks. Arrange on a serving dish around the dips.

Greek Salad

(Serves 4)

½ cucumber, thickly sliced
1 small onion, sliced
4 large tomatoes, sliced
4 black olives
100 g (4 oz) feta cheese, drained and cut into squares
4 tbsp olive oil
1 tbsp lemon juice
2 tsp chopped fresh oregano
½ small iceberg lettuce, shredded

1. Cut the cucumber slices into quarters and place in a bowl with the onion, tomatoes, olives and cheese. Mix well.
2. Combine the oil, lemon juice and oregano and blend together thoroughly. Place the lettuce in a glass bowl and spoon the salad ingredients on top. Pour the dressing over.

Oriental Rice Salad

(Serves 4)

150 g (6 oz) long grain white/brown rice
150 g (6 oz) basmati rice
1 tbsp sunflower oil
6 spring onions, finely chopped
1 courgette, thinly sliced lengthways
1 red pepper, thinly sliced lengthways
1 yellow pepper, thinly sliced lengthways
50 g (2 oz) mangetout
100 g (4 oz) beansprouts

2 tbsp tamari sauce
black pepper
lemon juice

1. Cook the rice in boiling water for 12–15 minutes until tender. Drain, rinse with boiling water, drain again, and set aside.
2. Heat the oil in a frying pan and add the onions, courgette, peppers, mangetout and beansprouts. Cook until just tender and slightly browned.
3. Add the tamari sauce, black pepper and lemon juice to the cooked rice. Continue cooking until all the grains are evenly coated.
4. Serve either hot or cold.

Variation: For a more substantial salad, add chicken or prawns.

Pepper and Lentil Salad

(Serves 4)
1 large red pepper, seeded and chopped
1 large green pepper, seeded and chopped
1 onion, finely chopped
10 pitted black olives, halved
1 tbsp chopped fresh thyme
50 g (2 oz) Puy lentils, cooked
4 tbsp olive oil
4 tbsp lemon juice
1 garlic clove, crushed
black pepper to taste

1. In a large bowl, mix together the red pepper, green pepper, onion, olives, thyme and lentils.
2. Whisk the oil, lemon, garlic and black pepper together and pour on to the lentil mixture. Mix well to coat all the ingredients.

Salad Niçoise

(Serves 4)
4 medium potatoes, scrubbed
4 medium tomatoes, cut into wedges
200 g (7 oz) can tuna in olive oil, drained and flaked
1 small crisp lettuce, separated into leaves
black pepper to taste
3 hard-boiled eggs, shelled and cut into wedges
50 g (2 oz) can anchovies in oil, drained
10 black olives
olive oil dressing, home-made or shop bought

1. Cook the potatoes in boiling, salted water for 15–20 minutes or until tender. Drain, cool, then cut into bite-sized pieces.
2. Mix the potato, tomatoes and tuna together.
3. Arrange the lettuce on a serving platter and spoon the tuna mixture into the middle. Sprinkle with black pepper.
4. Arrange the egg, anchovies and olives on top of the salad and pour over the olive oil dressing.

Seafood Salad

(Serves 4)
350 g (12 oz) cod fillet
½ white cabbage, trimmed
225 g (8 oz) peeled prawns
100 g (4 oz) cooked mussels, shelled
1 onion, grated
100 g (4 oz) carrots, grated
½ tsp chopped fresh dill
olive oil dressing, shop bought or home-made

1. Steam the cod until tender, then remove the skin and flake the fish. Leave to cool.
2. Shred the cabbage finely, then rinse and drain well. Pat dry with a clean cloth or kitchen paper.

3. Mix the cod, cabbage, prawns, mussels, onions, carrots and dill together.

4. Toss the salad in the olive oil dressing.

Spinach and Avocado Salad

(Serves 4)
40 English spinach leaves
200 g (7 oz) avocado, sliced
12 black olives, stoned and quartered

Dressing
10 ml (2 tsp) olive oil
15 ml (1 tbsp) lemon juice (fresh)
1 garlic clove, crushed

1. Remove the thick stalks from the spinach leaves and slice the leaves into bite-sized pieces.

2. Combine the spinach, avocado and olives in a bowl.

3. Combine the oil, lemon juice and garlic and pour this dressing over the salad.

Stuffed Peppers

(Serves 4)
4 medium green peppers
225 g (8 oz) cooked brown rice
2 apples, chopped
225 g (8 oz) canned sweetcorn
225 g (8 oz) carrot, shredded

1. Halve the peppers lengthways, scoop out the seeds and steam for 10 minutes.

2. Mix other ingredients together and use to stuff peppers.

3. Place in an oven-proof dish, cover and cook for 15 minutes at 200°C/400°F/Gas mark 6.

Tuna Jackets

(Serves 4)
15 ml (1 tbsp) sunflower oil
1 red, 1 yellow and 1 green pepper, cored, seeded and diced
60 ml (4 tbsp) white wine vinegar
30 ml (2 tbsp) wholegrain mustard
200 g (7 oz) can tuna in oil, drained and flaked
125 g (4 oz) can sweetcorn, drained
4 hot baked potatoes
freshly ground black pepper

1. Heat the oil, add the diced peppers and sauté for 5 minutes. Add the vinegar and mustard and cook for 5 minutes, stirring.
2. Stir in the flaked tuna and sweetcorn.
3. Cut the tops off the potatoes and scoop out the centres.
4. Chop the potato and stir it into half the pepper relish mixture. Season with black pepper to taste.
5. Spoon the potato mixture back into the potato jackets.
6. Serve the remaining relish separately.

SIDE SALADS

Bean and Sweetcorn Salad

(Serves 4)
225 g (8 oz) French beans, cooked, cooled and cut into 2.5-cm (1-in) lengths
100 g (4 oz) can of sweetcorn, drained
2 small spring onions
sesame seeds to garnish

1. Mix all the ingredients together with black pepper and dressing to taste.

Bean Salad

(Serves 4)
100 g (4 oz) haricot beans (soaked overnight)
100 g (4 oz) chickpeas (soaked overnight)
1 bay leaf
2 sprigs of thyme
1 clove garlic, crushed (optional)
100 g (4 oz) broad beans
100 g (4 oz) red kidney beans (canned)
1 medium onion, finely chopped
½ tsp cumin seeds, ground
2 tbsp (30 ml) cold-pressed olive or vegetable oil

1. Drain the haricot beans and chickpeas, and cover with water in a saucepan. Boil for 10 minutes, then add the bay leaf and sprigs of thyme, and simmer for 1 to 1½ hours. Drain and leave to cool.
2. Chop the onion.
3. Mix the garlic with the oil and kidney and broad beans. Pour over the remaining beans and sprinkle with the cumin seeds.

Beansprout Salad

(Serves 4)
175 g (6 oz) beansprouts
100 g (4 oz) red pepper, cored, seeded and sliced
100 g (4 oz) can sweetcorn, drained
2 dessert apples, grated
4 spring onions, chopped

1. Mix all the ingredients together with black pepper and dressing to taste.

Beetroot and Cabbage Salad

(Serves 4)

175 g (6 oz) firm white cabbage, shredded

175 g (6 oz) red cabbage, grated

175 g (6 oz) carrots, grated

1 small onion, finely chopped

½ red pepper, cored, seeded and chopped

25 g (1 oz) sunflower seeds

175 g (6 oz) raw beetroot, grated

1. Mix together all the ingredients, leaving the beetroot until just before serving.

Coleslaw

(Serves 4)

450 g (1 lb) white cabbage, shredded

100 g (4 oz) carrots, grated

1 small onion, sliced

2 tbsp low-fat mayonnaise or dressing or natural low-fat yogurt

1 tbsp finely chopped fresh parsley to garnish

1. Mix all ingredients together and place in a bowl.

Cauliflower and Carrot Salad

(Serves 4)

225 g (8 oz) raw carrot, cut into small sticks

225 g (8 oz) raw cauliflower, cut into small sprigs

225 g (8 oz) chopped cucumber

1 level tsp mixed herbs

1. Mix all ingredients together and place in a bowl.

Courgette and Cauliflower Salad

(Serves 4)

75 g (3 oz) courgettes, thinly sliced
225 g (8 oz) cauliflower, cut into small florets
100 g (4 oz) red pepper, cored and chopped
1 tsp freshly chopped fennel to garnish

1. Mix all ingredients together and place in a bowl.

Fruity Cabbage Salad

(Serves 4)

450 g (1 lb) white cabbage, shredded
100 g (4 oz) green pepper, chopped
5 radishes, sliced
1 red and 1 green apple, chopped
1 medium orange, broken into segments and halved
100 g (4 oz) chopped melon

1. Mix all ingredients together and place in a bowl.

Ginger and Carrot Salad

(Serves 4)

170 g (6 oz) carrots, grated
2 medium apples, grated
1 tsp ground ginger
1 stick of celery, chopped

1. Mix all ingredients together and place in a bowl.

Green Salad

(Serves 4)
225 g (8 oz) lettuce
8 slices thinly cut cucumber per portion
2 green peppers, cored, seeded and chopped
225 g (8 oz) watercress

1. Mix all ingredients together and place in a bowl.

Minty Cabbage Salad

(Serves 4)
250 g (9 oz) white cabbage
1 medium carrot
1 medium green pepper, cored and seeded
1 medium red pepper, cored and seeded
1 large bunch of fresh mint, chopped

1. Shred the cabbage, grate the carrot, chop the peppers and mix all the ingredients together.

Root Salad

(Serves 4)
100 g (4 oz) celeriac root
170 g (6 oz) carrots
100 g (4 oz) parsnip
75 g (3 oz) beetroot

1. Chop or grate the celeriac, carrots and parsnip, and mix together.
2. Chop beetroot and sprinkle on top of the salad.

Salad

s 4)

(8 oz) lettuce

s thinly cut cucumber per portion

n peppers, cored, seeded and chopped

(8 oz) watercress

ll ingredients together and place in a bowl.

Cabbage Salad

s 4)

(9 oz) white cabbage

ium carrot

ium green pepper, cored and seeded

ium red pepper, cored and seeded

bunch of fresh mint, chopped

the cabbage, grate the carrot, chop the peppers and mix all

gredients together.

alad

s 4)

(4 oz) celeriac root

(6 oz) carrots

4 oz) parsnip

oz) beetroot

or grate the celeriac, carrots and parsnip, and mix

er.

beetroot and sprinkle on top of the salad.

Bean Salad

(Serves 4)

100 g (4 oz) haricot beans (soaked overnight)

100 g (4 oz) chickpeas (soaked overnight)

1 bay leaf

2 sprigs of thyme

1 clove garlic, crushed (optional)

100 g (4 oz) broad beans

100 g (4 oz) red kidney beans (canned)

1 medium onion, finely chopped

½ tsp cumin seeds, ground

2 tbsp (30 ml) cold-pressed olive or vegetable oil

1. Drain the haricot beans and chickpeas, and cover with water in a saucepan. Boil for 10 minutes, then add the bay leaf and sprigs of thyme, and simmer for 1 to 1½ hours. Drain and leave to cool.
2. Chop the onion.
3. Mix the garlic with the oil and kidney and broad beans. Pour over the remaining beans and sprinkle with the cumin seeds.

Beansprout Salad

(Serves 4)

175 g (6 oz) beansprouts

100 g (4 oz) red pepper, cored, seeded and sliced

100 g (4 oz) can sweetcorn, drained

2 dessert apples, grated

4 spring onions, chopped

1. Mix all the ingredients together with black pepper and dressing to taste.

Beetroot and Cabbage Salad

(Serves 4)

175 g (6 oz) firm white cabbage, shredded
175 g (6 oz) red cabbage, grated
175 g (6 oz) carrots, grated
1 small onion, finely chopped
½ red pepper, cored, seeded and chopped
25 g (1 oz) sunflower seeds
175 g (6 oz) raw beetroot, grated

1. Mix together all the ingredients, leaving the beetroot until just before serving.

Coleslaw

(Serves 4)

450 g (1 lb) white cabbage, shredded
100 g (4 oz) carrots, grated
1 small onion, sliced
2 tbsp low-fat mayonnaise or dressing or natural low-fat yogurt
1 tbsp finely chopped fresh parsley to garnish

1. Mix all ingredients together and place in a bowl.

Cauliflower and Carrot Salad

(Serves 4)

225 g (8 oz) raw carrot, cut into small sticks
225 g (8 oz) raw cauliflower, cut into small sprigs
225 g (8 oz) chopped cucumber
1 level tsp mixed herbs

1. Mix all ingredients together and place in a bowl.

Courgette and Cauliflower Sal[

(Serves 4)

75 g (3 oz) courgettes, thinly sliced
225 g (8 oz) cauliflower, cut into small flore
100 g (4 oz) red pepper, cored and chopped
1 tsp freshly chopped fennel to garnish

1. Mix all ingredients together and place i[

Fruity Cabbage Salad

(Serves 4)

450 g (1 lb) white cabbage, shredded
100 g (4 oz) green pepper, chopped
5 radishes, sliced
1 red and 1 green apple, chopped
1 medium orange, broken into segments a[
100 g (4 oz) chopped melon

1. Mix all ingredients together and place i[

Ginger and Carrot Salad

(Serves 4)

170 g (6 oz) carrots, grated
2 medium apples, grated
1 tsp ground ginger
1 stick of celery, chopped

1. Mix all ingredients together and place [

Gree[

(Ser[

225 [
8 slic[
2 gre[
225 [

1. Mix [

Minty[

(Serv[

250 [
1 me[
1 me[
1 me[
1 larg[

1. Shre[
the i[

Root [

(Serv[

100 [
170 [
100 [
75 g [

1. Chop[
toget[
2. Chop[

Tomato and Celery Salad

(Serves 4)
225 g (8 oz) tomatoes, cut into 8 pieces
100 g (4 oz) celery, chopped
100g (4 oz) green pepper, finely sliced
100 g (4 oz) lettuce, shredded
1 tbsp freshly chopped parsley to garnish

1. Mix all ingredients together and place in a bowl.

Vege Salad

(Serves 4)
100 g (4 oz) courgettes, thinly sliced
75 g (3 oz) carrots, grated
75 g (3 oz) baby turnips, grated
50 g (2 oz) spinach leaves, coarsely chopped
225 g (8 oz) broad beans

1. Mix all the ingredients together with black pepper and dressing of choice to taste.

Waldorf Salad

(Serves 4)
50 g (2 oz) walnuts
1 head curly endive
2 dessert apples
2 sticks celery
1 tbsp linseeds
freshly ground black pepper

1. Chop the walnuts, endives, apples and celery, add the linseeds, and mix together.
2. Season with black pepper and dressing of your choice.

Watercress, Fennel and Lemon Salad

(Serves 4)

1 large fennel bulb, thinly sliced
1 small bunch watercress, washed and trimmed
1 handful parsley, washed, well dried and finely chopped
freshly ground black pepper
1 tbsp lemon juice (fresh)
1 lemon

1. Mix together the fennel, watercress and parsley.
2. Add the black pepper and lemon juice.
3. Thinly slice the lemon, cut each slice into segments and add to the salad.

DRESSINGS

Orange and Herb Sauce

(Serves 4)

10 ml (2 tsp) sunflower oil
1 small onion, finely chopped
175 ml (6 fl oz) fresh orange juice
2 tsp chopped tarragon
2 tsp chopped parsley
freshly ground black pepper
2 tsp cornflour
15 ml (1 tbsp) water
1 orange, peeled, segmented, pith removed and chopped

1. Heat the oil gently and fry the onion. Add the orange juice, herbs and black pepper.
2. Bring to the boil and simmer for 2–4 minutes.
3. Mix the cornflour with the water and stir into the sauce, bringing slowly to the boil and stirring constantly.

4. Add the chopped orange segments, heat for 1–2 minutes and serve.

This sauce can be used to complement meat, fish or vegetable dishes, and can be made in larger quantities in advance and frozen.

Spicy Lentil Dressing

(Serves 4)
225 g (8 oz) red lentils
600 ml (1 pint) water
10 ml (2 tsp) sunflower oil
1 onion, finely chopped
1 garlic clove, crushed
½ tsp ginger (ground or grated root)
½ tsp ground coriander
½ tsp ground cumin seeds

1. Place the lentils in a saucepan and cover with the measured water.
2. Bring to the boil and simmer for 20–30 minutes until the water has been absorbed and the lentils are swollen. The lentils should look like a thickish purée.
3. Heat the oil and gently fry the onions, garlic and ginger until lightly brown, for 4–6 minutes.
4. Add the spices and cook further for 1–2 minutes.
5. Add the lentils and cook very gently for 4–5 minutes. Serve hot with rice, or cold with salad.

Tomato Dressing

(Serves 4 – 2 tbsp each)
10 ml (2 tsp) olive oil
100 g (4 oz) onion, finely chopped
1 garlic clove, crushed
400 g (14 oz) fresh ripe tomatoes chopped and skin removed, or
400 ml (14 oz) can plum tomatoes, drained and chopped
½ tsp mixed herbs or basil
freshly ground black pepper to taste

1. Heat the oil, adding the onion and garlic. Cover and cook gently for 5 minutes until the onion is soft.
2. Add the tomatoes and herbs. Cover and cook for 15 minutes.
3. Season with black pepper and cool.

DINNERS – STAGES 1 AND 2

Almond Trout

(Serves 4)
4 trout, cleaned, with heads and tails intact
freshly ground black pepper
juice of 1 lemon
25 g (1 oz) margarine
50 g (2 oz) flaked almonds
4 sprigs parsley to garnish

1. Season the fish with pepper and lemon juice.
2. Melt the margarine and lightly brush the fish with it.
3. Place the fish under a hot grill and cook for 6 minutes each side.
4. Brush one side again lightly with melted margarine and arrange almonds over the fish. Grill again for 1 minute or until the almonds start to brown.
5. Garnish with parsley and serve.

Beef Stroganoff

(Serves 4)

2 tsp oil
30 g (1 oz) butter
1 medium onion, finely sliced
100 g (4 oz) red pepper, chopped
½ beef stock cube
150 ml (¼ pint) boiling water
1 level tsp tomato purée
450 g (1 lb) fillet of beef cut into thin strips
6 level tbsp (90 ml) soured cream
freshly ground black pepper to taste

1. Heat half the oil and half the butter in a non-stick frying pan. Add the onion, and cook over a low heat, stirring frequently, until soft.
2. Stir in the peppers.
3. Dissolve the stock cube in the water, stir in the tomato purée, then add to the frying pan. Boil rapidly until the liquid is reduced to about 60 ml (4 tablespoons). Tip the reduced liquid into a bowl and set aside.
4. Heat the remaining oil and butter in the pan and add the meat, which should all fit in the pan easily in a single layer. If necessary, cook it in two batches. Cook over a fairly high heat until the outsides are browned – about 3 minutes each side. Shake and toss the pan frequently as the meat cooks. Add the vegetable mixture and heat through. Add the soured cream and season. Heat through but do not allow to boil.
5. Serve immediately.

Chicken with Almonds

(Serves 4)

4 chicken breasts
15 g (½ oz) butter or margarine
150 ml (¼ pint) water
a few black peppercorns
75 g (3 oz) flaked almonds

1. Skin the chicken and brush with melted butter or margarine.
2. Place water and peppercorns in an ovenprooof dish. Place the chicken in the water and cover with foil. Bake for 15 minutes in a preheated oven at 180°C/350°F/Gas mark 4.
3. Remove the foil and sprinkle with flaked almonds. Return to the oven for a further 15 minutes, or until the chicken is tender and the almonds have browned.
4. Serve with steamed vegetables, eg new potatoes and broccoli.

Chicken with Peach Sauce

(Serves 4)

1.6 kg (3½ lb) fresh chicken, skinned and cut into pieces
freshly ground black pepper
2 tbsp vegetable oil
1 small onion, finely chopped
1 garlic clove, crushed
¼ tsp red pepper flakes
½ tsp ground ginger
250 ml (8 fl oz) vegetable stock
50 ml (2 fl oz) lime juice
50 ml (2 fl oz) lemon juice
1 tbsp sunflower oil
4 fresh peaches, halved, stoned and sliced

1. Preheat the oven to 190°C/375°F/Gas mark 5.
2. Sprinkle the black pepper over the chicken pieces and set them aside.

3. In a large frying pan heat the oil and add the chicken pieces a few at a time. Fry, turning occasionally, for 8–10 minutes. With a slotted spoon, remove the chicken from the pan and transfer to a medium-sized ovenproof casserole.

4. Add the onion and garlic to the pan and fry them, stirring occasionally, for 5–7 minutes or until the onion is soft and translucent but not brown.

5. Stir in the pepper flakes, ginger and stock, and bring the mixture to the boil, stirring constantly.

6. Remove the pan from the heat and stir in the lime and lemon juices. Pour the mixture over the chicken pieces in the casserole. Set aside.

7. Melt the oil in a clean frying pan and gently fry the peaches for 6 minutes, or until they begin to turn to pulp. Transfer from the pan to the casserole dish.

Chilli & Corn Fritters with Scrambled Eggs

(Serves 4)
1 cup (150 g) plain flour
1 tsp baking powder
Salt & freshly ground black pepper
2 corn cobs (or 1 cup corn niblets, drained, rinsed)
1 small red chilli, finely chopped
2 eggs
½ cup (125 ml) soya milk
2 tbsps vegetable oil
30 g (1 oz) baby spinach leaves, to serve
6 roma tomatoes, halved, grilled
6 slices prosciutto, grilled

Scrambled Egg
4 eggs
¼ cup (60 ml) soya milk
30 g butter

1. Sift the flour and baking powder into a large bowl. Season with salt and pepper. If using fresh corn, use a sharp knife to cut the corn kernels from the cobs. Add corn, chilli, eggs and soya milk to the flour mixture. Mix to form a stiff batter.

2. Heat the oil in a non-stick frying pan and add 2 tablespoons of batter for each fritter. Cook for 2 minutes each side or until golden brown and cooked through. Drain on paper towel. Repeat until all the batter is used.

3. To make the scrambled eggs, whisk the eggs and soya milk together. Season with salt and pepper. Heat the butter in a non-stick frying pan until foaming. Add the egg mixture and cook over low heat, using a wooden spoon to move the mixture gently around the pan, for 2–3 minutes or until just set.

4. Serve the scrambled eggs, spinach, tomato and prosciutto sandwiched between two fritters.

Cumin Chicken

(Serves 4)
2 tsp vegetable oil
2 tsp cumin seeds
4 × 100g (4 oz) chicken breast fillets, cubed
1 red pepper, chopped
6 spring onions, chopped
2 tsp finely chopped root ginger
600 ml (1 pint) of stock
cornflour
water

1. Heat the oil in saucepan, add the cumin seeds and stir until they start popping.

2. Add chicken, pepper, onions and ginger; stir for 3 minutes.

3. Add the stock, bring to the boil, simmer for 5 minutes.

4. Add the cornflour (mixed into paste with cold water), and simmer for a further 5 minutes before serving.

Fish Stew with Peppers

(Serves 4)

30 ml (2 tbsp) sunflower oil
450 g (1 lb) canned, peeled tomatoes
1 red chilli, seeded and finely chopped
2 green peppers, cored, seeded and sliced
2 medium onions, finely chopped
3 garlic cloves, crushed
50 ml (2 fl oz) dry white wine (avoid if on a yeast-free diet)
1 tsp dried thyme
1 bay leaf
900 g (2 lb) sole fillets, cut into 2.5 cm (1 in) cubes
450 g (1 lb) small new potatoes, scrubbed, cooked until just tender and kept warm

1. In an ovenproof dish heat the oil and add the tomatoes, including the juice, and the chilli. Stirring occasionally, cook for 15 minutes or until the mixture is thick.
2. Stir in the green peppers, onions, garlic, wine, thyme, bay leaf and fish cubes. Cover the dish, reduce the heat to low, and cook for 10 minutes, stirring occasionally.
3. Add the potatoes and turn them over in the fish mixture. Cover again and cook for a further 5 minutes, until the fish flakes easily when tested with a fork.
4. Discard the bay leaf and serve at once.

Green Chicken Curry

(Serves 6)

1 tbsp vegetable oil
500 g (1 lb) chicken tenderloins, diagonally cut into strips
2–3 tbsps (about 50 g) Thai green curry paste
140 ml can coconut cream
1 cup (250mL) soya milk
1 tbsp fish sauce
225 g (9 oz) can sliced bamboo shoots, drained, rinsed

125 g (5 oz) baby corn
100 g (4 oz) snow peas, trimmed
½ cup fresh Thai basil leaves
Steamed jasmine rice, to serve

1. Heat the oil in a wok. Add the chicken and curry paste, and cook over medium heat, stirring constantly for 5 minutes or until seared all over.
2. Add the coconut cream, Soya Milk and fish sauce and bring to the boil, stirring occasionally. Add bamboo shoots and corn and cook for 5 minutes or until corn is just tender.
3. Remove from heat and stir in snow peas and basil. Serve with rice.

Haddock Kedgeree

(Serves 4)
350 g (12 oz) unsmoked haddock, filleted and skinned
175 g (6 oz) brown rice
2 hard-boiled eggs, chopped
1 medium onion, finely chopped
1 green pepper, chopped
2 sprigs of parsley, chopped
4 tbsp low-fat natural yogurt
freshly ground black pepper to taste
4 slices of lemon

1. Cover the fish with water in a shallow pan. Heat gently and poach for about 8–10 minutes.
2. Remove the fish and flake.
3. Boil the rice in the poaching water left in the pan for about 10 minutes, checking the cooking instructions on the rice packet. You may need to add extra water.
4. Drain the rice, stir in the fish, egg, onion, pepper, parsley and yogurt and mix well. Heat gently, stirring all the time.
5. Season with pepper and serve garnished with lemon slices.

Halibut Fruit

(Serves 4)
finely grated rind and juice of 4 oranges
finely grated rind and juice of 2 lemons
4 halibut steaks, cut in half
2 oranges, peeled, segmented and skinned
orange and lemon slices to garnish

1. Preheat the oven to at 180°C/350°F/Gas mark 4.
2. Place the grated citrus rind in an ovenproof dish with the juices. Add the fish and baste well. This can be left to marinate for 1–6 hours, turning occasionally.
3. Cover the dish with foil and cook in the preheated oven for 10 minutes.
4. Add the orange segments and cook for a further 10 minutes.
5. Serve garnished with slices of lemon and orange.

Hot Fruity Chicken

(Serves 4)
2 tbsp concentrated apple juice
2 garlic cloves, chopped
4 tsp peeled grated ginger
4 tsp chilli sauce
600 g (1¼ lb) chicken breast, skinned and boned, and cut into strips
20 ml (4 tsp) sunflower oil
300 g (10 oz) onions, sliced
2 medium green peppers, cored, seeded and chopped
2 tsp cornflour
freshly ground black pepper
4 large oranges, peeled, segmented and skinned

1. Mix together the apple juice, half the garlic, the ginger and the chilli sauce. Add the chicken and coat thoroughly. Cover and refrigerate for at least 1 hour to marinate. It can be left overnight. Remove the chicken and reserve the marinade.

2. Heat the oil and sauté the onion and remaining garlic until the onion is translucent.

3. Add the chicken and chopped peppers and cook until the chicken is lightly browned on both sides.

4. Strain the reserved marinade and mix it with the cornflour.

5. Add the cornflour mixture and black pepper to taste to the pan. Bring to the boil, stirring constantly. Reduce the heat to a simmer.

6. Add the orange segments and heat through thoroughly, stirring occasionally. Serve immediately.

Japanese Sardines

(Serves 4)

100 ml (4 fl oz) tamari sauce
50 ml (2 floz) white wine or sherry vinegar
2 tbsp lemon juice
25 g (1 oz) fresh root ginger, peeled and chopped
2 garlic cloves, crushed
450 g (1 lb) fresh sardines, cleaned and washed thoroughly in cold water and dried

1. In a small mixing bowl, combine the tamari sauce, vinegar, lemon juice, ginger and garlic.

2. Arrange the sardines in a shallow baking dish and pour the tamari sauce mixture over them. Leave in a cool place to marinate for 1½–2 hours.

3. Remove the sardines from the marinade, and discard the marinade.

4. Grill for 3–5 minutes or longer, depending on the size, turning once. Serve immediately.

Lamb and Apricot Pilaff

(Serves 4)

2 tbsp sunflower oil
1 medium onion, thinly sliced
700 g (1½ lb) boned leg of lamb, cut into 2.5 cm (1 in) cubes
75 g (3 oz) dried apricots, soaked overnight, drained and halved
3 tbsp raisins
½ tsp ground cinnamon
freshly ground black pepper
900 ml (1½ pints) water
225 g (8 oz) long-grain rice, washed, soaked in cold water for 30 minutes and drained

1. Heat the oil in a frying pan, add the onion and cook for about 5 minutes, until translucent but not brown.
2. Add the lamb and cook, stirring and turning occasionally, for 5–8 minutes, or until lightly browned all over.
3. Stir in the apricots, raisins, cinnamon, pepper and half of the water. Bring to the boil, stirring occasionally. Reduce the heat to low, cover the pan and simmer for 1–1¼ hours, or until the meat is tender when pierced with the point of a sharp knife.
4. Cook the rice in the usual way, using the remaining water.
5. Preheat the oven to 180°C/350°F/Gas mark 4.
6. Place one-third of the meat in a medium casserole. Cover with a layer of one-third of the rice mixture, then top with another third of the meat. Continue to make the layers in this manner until all the ingredients have been used up, finishing with a layer of rice. Cover the casserole and bake for 50 minutes. Serve immediately.

Lamb in a Spicy Yogurt Sauce

(Serves 4)

225 ml (8 fl oz) water
15 ml (1 tbsp) olive oil
3 onions, sliced
900 g (2 lb) leg of lamb, boned and cut into 2 cm (¼ in) cubes
freshly ground black pepper
2 garlic cloves, crushed
1 tsp chopped fresh parsley
1 tsp sweet chilli sauce
600 ml (1 pint) yogurt
1 tbsp cornflour mixed to a paste with 10 ml (2 tsp) water
1 tsp grated lemon rind
1 tbsp chopped fresh coriander leaves (dried can be used)

1. In a large saucepan, bring the water and oil to the boil over a moderate heat.
2. Add the onions, lamb, pepper, garlic, chilli sauce and parsley. Cover the pan tightly, reduce the heat to low and simmer for 1¼ hours or until the lamb is very tender and the liquid has reduced by about two-thirds.
3. In a medium saucepan, heat the yogurt and cornflour mixture over a moderate heat, stirring constantly. Reduce the heat to very low and cook for 8 minutes or until it has reduced by half its original quantity.
4. Add the yogurt mixture and the lemon rind to the lamb mixture, stir well and simmer, uncovered, for 15 minutes.
5. Add the coriander and serve with a crisp salad and boiled rice.

Lamb Kebabs

(Serves 4)
450 g (1 lb) lamb neck fillet, trimmed and cut into chunks
1 green pepper
1 red pepper
1 large onion
450 g (1 lb) button mushrooms

Marinade
3 tbsp plain yogurt
juice ½ lime
2 garlic cloves, crushed
3 tbsp chopped fresh coriander
1 tbsp chopped fresh mint
1 tsp each curry powder and cumin
pinch each of salt and cayenne pepper

1. Combine the marinade ingredients in a large bowl. Add the lamb and stir. Cover and chill for at least 2 hours.
2. Thread the lamb, peppers, onions and mushrooms on to skewers in an alternate pattern. Cook for 4–6 minutes on each side (either on a barbecue on under a hot grill). Serve with lime wedges.

Mackerel with Lemon Stuffing

(Serves 4)
4 × 175 g (6 oz) mackerel, split and boned
juice of ½ lemon
freshly grated black pepper
3 tbsp water
4 slices lemon

Stuffing
2 tsp sunflower oil
1 small onion, finely chopped
125 g (4½ oz) cooked brown rice

finely grated rind and juice of ½ lemon
1 tbsp freshly chopped parsley
1 small egg, beaten

1. Preheat the oven to 160°C/325°F/Gas mark 3.
2. First prepare the stuffing. Heat the oil in the pan, add the onion and cook for 5 minutes or until golden brown. Transfer to a mixing bowl and combine with the remaining stuffing ingredients.
3. Place the mackerel on a flat surface and sprinkle the flesh with lemon juice and black pepper. Spoon the stuffing into the fish and reshape.
4. Place the fish in an ovenproof dish, and add the water. Cover and bake in the preheated oven for 15–20 minutes.
5. Serve immediately, garnished with the lemon slices.

Pizza Base

200 g (7 oz) plain flour
1 tsp baking powder
1 egg
75 ml (3 fl oz) milk
1 tbsp olive oil
1½ tbsp Sunflower oil

1. Mix the flour and baking powder together in a bowl.
2. Whist the egg, milk and oil together in another bowl.
3. Stir in the liquid and kneed it into a soft dough
4. Turn the dough on to a lightly oiled baking sheet or pizza dish and move into the desired shape with your fingers.
5. Add the toppings of your choice.

Poached Halibut with Parsley Sauce

(Serves 4)
1 small leek, chopped
1 carrot, chopped
2 tbsp freshly chopped parsley
4 halibut steaks
3 tbsp lemon juice
150 ml (5 fl oz) water

1. Place the chopped vegetables and 1 tablespoon of parsley over the bottom of a large pan. Add the steaks on top with the lemon juice and water.
2. Bring to the boil, cover and simmer for about 10 minutes. Transfer the halibut to a serving dish and keep warm.
3. Bring the liquid and vegetables back to the boil and simmer for a further 5 minutes.
4. Blend the vegetables to a purée and return to saucepan. Add the remaining tablespoon of parsley and reduce the liquid until it has thickened.
5. Pour this liquid over the halibut steaks and serve.

Prawn and Vegetable Stir-fry

(Serves 4)
3 tbsp (45 ml) vegetable oil
100 g (4 oz) broccoli, divided into florets
100 g (4 oz) carrots, cut into small, matchstick-sized pieces
100 g (4 oz) leeks, thinly sliced
225 g (8 oz) peeled prawns
50 g (2 oz) courgettes, thinly sliced
100 g (4 oz) Chinese leaves, roughly chopped
1 apple, cored and diced
1 tbsp grated ginger
100 g (4 oz) onions, chopped
1 tbsp (15 ml) lemon juice

1. Heat oil in a wok or large frying pan, add the broccoli, carrots and leeks and cook for 3 minutes.
2. Add the prawns, courgettes, Chinese leaves, apple, ginger, onions and lemon juice.
3. Stir-fry for a further 2 minutes.
4. Serve immediately.

Salmon and Cheese Roll

(Serves 4)
75 g (3 oz) cottage cheese
75 g (3 oz) curd cheese
2 tsp lemon juice
1 apple, shredded
black pepper to taste
8 × 30 g (1 oz) slices smoked salmon
4 lemon slices
100 g (4 oz) lettuce, chopped

1. Mix the cottage and curd cheese with the lemon juice and shredded apple. Season with black pepper.
2. Lay each smoked-salmon slice on a flat surface and spread with the cheese mixture. Roll up (like a Swiss roll).
3. Garnish with lemon slices and serve on a bed of lettuce.

Salmon Steaks with Ginger

(Serves 4)
4 salmon steaks
4 tbsp lemon juice
5 cm (2 in) square of fresh ginger, peeled and finely chopped
freshly ground black pepper to taste

1. Place each salmon steak on a large piece of foil. Add 1 tablespoon of lemon juice and a quarter of the chopped ginger to each steak. Season with a little black pepper.

2. Wrap the steaks individually in foil to make four parcels and bake in a preheated oven at 180°C/350°F/Gas mark 4 for 20 minutes. Serve hot with vegetables or cold with a salad.

Stuffed Mackerel

(Serves 4)

2 oranges
2 apples, grated
2 tbsp parsley, finely chopped
2 medium onions, finely chopped
4 tbsp cooked brown rice
4 × 140 g (5 oz) fresh mackerel, gutted
2 tsp dried rosemary or 8 sprigs fresh rosemary

1. Grate the peel of the oranges and chop flesh into small pieces, discarding pips.
2. Mix the oranges, apples, parsley, onions and rice together.
3. Divide mixture into four and use to stuff the mackerel loosely.
4. Place some rosemary in each fish.
5. Bake in foil for about 40 minutes at 200°C/400°F/Gas mark 6.

Sussex Casserole

(Serves 4)

900 g (2 lb) potatoes peeled and thickly sliced
900 g (2 lb) lean braising steak, cut into 2.5 cm (1 in) cubes
2 medium onions, peeled and finely chopped
6 sticks, celery, trimmed and chopped
450 g (1 lb) pickling onions
8 green olives, stoned
freshly ground black pepper to taste
1 tsp grated nutmeg
4 whole cloves (optional)
15 ml (1 tbsp) apple juice
450 ml (1 pint) vegetable stock
1 tbsp cornflour dissolved in water

1. Preheat the oven to 180°C/350°F/Gas mark 4.
2. Cover the bottom of an ovenproof casserole with half the potato slices.
3. Arrange half the steak cubes on top and cover with the onions, celery, pickling onions and olives. Sprinkle with black pepper and nutmeg.
4. Add the cloves (optional).
5. Cover with remaining steak and potatoes.
6. Mix together the apple juice, stock and cornflour mixture.
7. Pour over the meat, vegetables and potatoes. Cover and cook for 2½ hours. Remove the lid and increase the heat to 200°C/400°F/Gas mark 6 for a further 30 minutes, or until the potatoes are tender and golden brown. Remove from the oven, picking out the cloves (if used) and serve at once.

Turkey and Chickpeas with Rice

(Serves 4)

50 g (2 oz) margarine
12 pickling onions
900 g (2 lb) turkey breast, cut into 2.5 cm (1 in) cubes
100 g (4 oz) chickpeas, soaked overnight and drained
225 ml (8 fl oz) vegetable stock
freshly ground black pepper
1 tsp cumin seeds
pinch of turmeric
450 g (1 lb) long-grain rice, washed, soaked in cold water for 30 minutes and drained

1. Melt the margarine in a large pan over a moderate heat. Add the onions and turkey cubes and cook, stirring and turning, 5–8 minutes, until the onions are golden.
2. Add the chickpeas, stock and enough water to cover the mixture completely.
3. Add the pepper to taste, cumin and turmeric to the pan and stir

well to blend. Cover the pan and cook for 1¼ hours or until the turkey and chickpeas are tender.

4. Raise the heat and bring the liquid to the boil. Stir in the rice. Cover the pan, reduce the heat and simmer for 15–20 minutes or until the rice is tender and the liquid absorbed.

5. Remove the pan from the heat, spoon the mixture into a warmed serving dish and serve immediately.

Turkey Schnitzel

(Serves 4)
3 tbsp plain flour
seasoning
1 large egg, beaten
50 g (2 oz) fresh white breadcrumbs
4 × 175 g (6 oz) turkey breast escalopes

1. Sprinkle the flour on to a plate and season with a little salt and lots of black pepper. Pour the beaten egg on to another plate, and sprinkle the breadcrumbs on to a third plate.

2. Coat each escalope with the seasoned flour. Dip each floured escalope into the beaten egg, then dip into the breadcrumbs.

3. Cover and leave in the refrigerator for 30 minutes.

4. Bake in the oven for 30–40 minutes at 180°C/350°F/Gas mark 4 until the turkey is cooked through and the breadcrumbs are golden brown.

VEGETARIAN LUNCHES AND DINNERS – STAGE 1

Bean and Tomato Hotpot

(Serves 4)
30 ml (2 tbsp) sunflower oil
2 onions, sliced
3 carrots, sliced
2 sticks celery, sliced
1 large leek, sliced
2 garlic cloves, crushed
415 g (15 oz) can red kidney beans, drained
400 g (14 oz) can tomatoes
300 ml (½ pint) stock
1 tbsp yeast extract
freshly ground black pepper
750 g (1½ lb) potatoes, thinly sliced
15 g (½ oz) margarine

1. Preheat the oven to 180°C/350°F/Gas mark 4.
2. Heat the oil in a flameproof casserole, add the onions and fry for 5 minutes. Add the carrots, celery, leek and garlic and fry for a further 5 minutes.
3. Add the kidney beans, tomatoes with their juice, stock, yeast extract and pepper to taste. Mix well.
4. Arrange the potatoes in layers neatly on top, sprinkling pepper between each layer. Dot with margarine, cover and cook in the oven for 2 hours.
5. Remove the lid 30 minutes before the end of cooking to allow the potatoes to brown.

Herb Tofu

(Serves 4)
1 dessertspoon vegetable oil
1 small red pepper, cored, seeded and thinly sliced
1 garlic clove, crushed
175 g (6 oz) tofu, cubed
½ tbsp chopped parsley

1. Heat the oil in a frying pan.
2. Add the red pepper and garlic and fry for 2–3 minutes.
3. Add the tofu and parsley and continue to stir-fry until the tofu is heated through. Serve immediately.

Mexican Omelette

(Makes 2)
6 eggs
2 tbsp water
2 tbsp oil

Filling
1 tbsp olive oil
1 onion, finely chopped
1 garlic clove, finely crushed
1 green pepper, cored and finely chopped
2 ripe tomatoes, peeled, seeded and chopped
125 g (4 oz) button mushrooms, thinly sliced
225 g tin spicy mixed beans*

*Check the labels and buy a brand which does not contain modified starch

1. Make the filling. heat the oil in a frying pan, add the onion and garlic and cook for 5 minutes or until softened. Add the pepper, and cook, stirring, for 5 minutes.

2. Add the tomatoes and mushrooms, and cook stirring, for 10 minutes. Add the tin of mixed beans, salt and pepper to taste and simmer for 5 minutes. Keep warm.

3. Beat 3 of the eggs with 1 tbsp of the measured water. Heat half of the oil in the frying pan.

4. When the oil is hot enough add the eggs, cooking over a medium heat, pulling back the edge as the eggs set, tilting the pan to allow the uncooked egg to run to the side of the pan. Continue until slightly set and golden.

5. Spoon half of the filling on to the half of the omelette farthest away from the pan handle. With a palette knife, lift the uncovered half of the omelette and flip it over the filling.

6. Slide the omelette on to a warmed plate. Make the second omelette in the same way.

Mexican Stuffed Eggs

(Serves 4)
4 hard-boiled eggs
1 medium avocado, peeled, stoned and chopped
1 small onion, finely minced
1 small green pepper, cored, seeded and finely minced
100 g (4 oz) prawns or shrimps, shelled, deveined and finely chopped, or almond halves, finely chopped
5 ml (1 tsp) lemon juice
5 ml (1 tsp) wine vinegar
freshly ground black pepper to taste
1 pinch of cayenne pepper
1 tbsp chopped parsley

1. Slice the eggs in half lengthways and scoop out the yolks. Set the whites aside. Using the back of a wooden spoon rub the yolks and the avocado flesh through a fine nylon strainer into a medium-sized mixing bowl. Stir in the onion, green pepper and chopped prawns or nuts.

2. Add the lemon juice, vinegar, pepper and cayenne, mixing well to blend.

3. With a teaspoon, generously stuff the egg-white halves with the mixture. Arrange on a serving dish, sprinkle with parsley and chill well before serving.

Mixed Vegetable and Almond Stir-fry

(Serves 4)
450 g (1 lb) fresh broccoli
225 g (8 oz) cauliflower
1 tbsp oil
2.5 cm (1 in) fresh root ginger, sliced and finely shredded
100 g (4 oz) flaked almonds
2 large carrots, peeled and sliced
½ tsp sesame oil
225 g (8 oz) fresh beansprouts
225 g (8 oz) Chinese leaves or white cabbage, shredded
½ tsp salt

1. Separate the broccoli heads into small florets and peel and slice the stems. Separate the cauliflower florets and slice stems.

2. Heat the oil in a large wok or frying pan. When it is moderately hot, add ginger shreds. Stir-fry for a few seconds, then add the almonds and stir-fry until they are gently browned.

3. Add the carrots, cauliflower and broccoli and stir-fry 2–3 minutes, then add the sesame oil.

4. Add the beansprouts and Chinese leaves, and stir-fry for about 5 minutes.

5. Serve with noodles or rice.

Nut and Vegetable Loaf

(Serves a generous 4)
10 ml (2 tsp) sunflower oil
1 small onion, chopped
1 small carrot, chopped
1 stick celery, chopped
15 ml (1 tbsp) tomato purée
225 g (8 oz) tomatoes, skinned and chopped
2 eggs
1 tbsp chopped parsley
freshly ground black pepper
225 g (8 oz) mixed nuts, finely chopped, or minced

To garnish
onion rings
parsley sprigs

1. Preheat the oven to 220°C/425°F/Gas mark 7.
2. Melt the oil in a pan, add the onion, carrot and celery and cook until softened. Add the tomato purée and tomatoes and cook for 5 minutes.
3. Put the eggs, parsley and pepper to taste in a bowl and beat well. Stir in the nuts and vegetables.
4. Transfer to a greased 900 ml (1½ pint) ovenproof dish and bake 30–35 minutes.
5. Turn out and decorate with onion rings and parsley. Serve hot with vegetables and sauce, or cold with salad.

Nutty Quorn Risotto

(Serves 4)
225 g (8 oz) brown rice
1 tbsp (15 ml) sunflower oil
1 medium onion
1 clove garlic
1 red pepper, seeded and sliced

1 green pepper, seeded and sliced
50 g (2 oz) green beans
100 g (4 oz) carrots, cut into matchsticks
100 g (4 oz) courgettes, thinly sliced
100 g (4 oz) broccoli, broken into florets and with stalks sliced
225 g (8 oz) Quorn
1 small seedless orange, broken into segments and skin removed
1 tbsp flaked almonds
1 tbsp of fresh chopped parsley

1. Cook the rice as directed on the packet and put to one side.
2. Heat the oil in a large frying pan. Add the onion, garlic, red and green peppers and gently fry for 2–3 minutes.
3. Steam the beans, carrots, courgettes and broccoli over a pan of boiling water for 5 minutes (or add them straight to the pan if you like your vegetables crunchy), then add to the other ingredients in the frying pan.
4. Add the Quorn, orange, flaked almonds, parsley and rice and heat through until all the ingredients are hot. Serve immediately.

Nutty Sprout Stir-fry

(Serves 4)
75 g (3 oz) unsalted peanuts
1 medium orange, peeled and cut into segments
10 ml (2 tsp) oil
1 pinch of cayenne
½ tsp ground cumin seeds
2 thick spring onions, trimmed and sliced
1 garlic clove, thinly sliced
175 g (6 oz) Brussels sprouts, trimmed and thinly sliced
1 red pepper, cored, seeded and thinly sliced
30 ml (2 tbsp) wheat-free soy or tamari sauce

1. Place the peanuts on a baking dish in a pre-heated oven (190°C/ 375°F/Gas mark 5) until they are lightly roasted.
2. Slice the orange segments crossways into triangles.
3. Heat the oil in a wok or heavy frying pan. Add the cayenne, cumin, spring onions, garlic and sprouts and toss in the oil for 1 minute.
4. Add the roasted peanuts and red pepper, mix and fry again for 1 minute.
5. Lastly, add the orange triangles and soy sauce and stir-fry until all the vegetables are coated and the oranges are heated through. Serve immediately.

Polenta with Grilled Vegetables

(Serves 4–6)
175 g (6 oz) polenta
150 ml (¼ pint) cold water
600 ml (1 pint) boiling water
30 g (1 oz) butter
2 courgettes, halved and thickly sliced lengthways
1 fennel bulb, trimmed and quartered lengthways
2 tomatoes, cored and sliced
1 aubergine, halved and sliced lengthways
1 red pepper, halved and sliced
1 green pepper, halved and sliced

Marinade 1
2 tbsp olive oil
2 tbsp red wine vinegar
2–3 tbsp chopped parsley
2 garlic cloves, crushed
salt and black pepper

1. Put the polenta into a saucepan, cover with the measured cold water, and leave to stand for 5 minutes.
2. Add the boiling salted water to the pan, return to the boil, and simmer for 10–15 minutes, stirring until smooth and thickened.

3. Sprinkle a baking tray with water. Stir the butter into the polenta; then spread the mixture over the tray in a 1 cm (½ in) layer. Leave to cool.

4. Make the marinade: combine the oil, vinegar, parsley, garlic and salt and pepper. Add the vegetables and leave to marinate in the refrigerator for 30 minutes.

5. Lift the vegetables out of the marinade and cook over a hot barbecue (or under a grill) for 2–3 minutes on each side. Cut the polenta into strips and cook over a barbecue (or grill), brushing with melted butter, for 1–2 minutes on each side until golden. Serve hot.

Variation: To adapt this recipe, use marinade 2.

Marinade 2
2 tbsp sunflower oil
2 tbsp tamari sauce (wheat-free soya sauce)
1 tbsp clear honey
2 tsp Dijon mustard
salt and black pepper

Red Lentil and Coconut Smoothie

(Serves 4)
225 g (8 oz) red split lentils
100 g (4 oz) carrots, sliced
1 medium onion, finely chopped
1 clove of garlic, crushed
1 tsp of paprika
½ tsp of ground ginger
1 bay leaf
15 g (½ oz) creamed coconut, finely chopped
2 tbsp lemon juice
black pepper to taste

1. Wash the lentils and put into a large saucepan with carrots, onion, garlic, paprika, ginger, bay leaf and 600 ml (1 pint) of water. Bring

to the boil, remove any scum, cover the pan and simmer 25–30 minutes until the water has been absorbed.

2. Remove the bay leaf and mash the mixture into a smooth paste with a fork. Add the coconut, lemon juice and black pepper.

3. Serve hot with vegetables or rice.

Root Veggie Bake

(Serves 4)
450 g (1 lb) potatoes, scrubbed and sliced
340 g (12 oz) parsnips and carrots, scrubbed and sliced
1 tbsp chopped peanuts
1 tbsp of fresh parsley, chopped
tomato sauce (see below)
Cheddar cheese, grated

Tomato sauce
2 tsp olive oil
100 g (4 oz) onion, finely chopped
1 clove garlic, crushed
385 g (14 oz) fresh ripe tomatoes, chopped and skin removed, or 1 can (385 g/14 oz) plum tomatoes, drained and chopped
good pinch mixed herbs or basil
freshly ground black pepper to taste

1. For the sauce, heat the oil, add the onion and garlic, cover, and cook gently for 5 minutes until the onion is soft.

2. Add the tomatoes and herbs. Cover and cook for 15 minutes.

3. Season with fresh pepper.

4. Bring the potatoes, carrots and parsnips to the boil in a pan of water and simmer for 10 minutes then drain.

5. Grease a large ovenproof dish. Layer the potatoes, carrots, parsnips with the nuts, parsley and the tomato sauce.

6. Sprinkle the top with cheese and bake in a pre heated oven at 180°C/350°F/Gas mark 4 for 15 minutes. Serve immediately.

Spanish Rice

(Serves 4)

45 ml (3 tbsp) olive oil
2 onions, thinly sliced
2 garlic cloves, crushed
1 green pepper, cored, seeded and thinly sliced
2 red peppers, cored, seeded and thinly sliced
350 g (12 oz) mushrooms, thinly sliced
400 g (14 oz) canned, chopped tomatoes
40 g (1½ oz) stoned green olives (optional)
1 tsp dried oregano
½ tsp basil
freshly ground black pepper to taste
150 g (5 oz) cooked rice

1. Heat the oil in a large frying pan. Add the onions and garlic and cook for 5–7 minutes, stirring occasionally.
2. Add the green and red peppers and cook for 4 minutes, stirring frequently. Add the mushrooms, tomatoes with their juice, olives, oregano, basil and black pepper to the pan and cook, stirring occasionally, for 3 minutes.
3. Add the rice to the pan and cook for 3–4 minutes, stirring constantly until the rice is heated through.
4. Serve immediately as a hot dish but equally good cold.

Vegetable Curry

(Serves 4)

4 tsp vegetable oil
2 garlic cloves, crushed
½ tsp turmeric
½ tsp ground coriander
½ tsp cumin seeds
2 tsp finely chopped ginger

1 small chilli, seeded and finely chopped
350 g (12 oz) boiled butter beans
175 g (6 oz) cauliflower, broken into florets
175 g (6 oz) turnip, cut into 2.5 cm (1 in) cubes
175 g (6 oz) parsnip, cut into 2.5 cm (1 in) cubes
175 g (6 oz) courgettes, thickly sliced
1 small onion, chopped
4 tbsp tomato purée
1.75 litres (3 pints) vegetable stock

1. Heat the oil in a large saucepan. Add garlic, spices and chilli and stir over a moderate heat for 2 minutes.
2. Add all remaining ingredients, mix well and bring to the boil.
3. Cover and simmer for 15 minutes, then for a further 10 minutes without a lid.
4. Serve with brown rice and small salad.

VEGETARIAN LUNCHES AND DINNERS – STAGE 2

Frittata

(Serves 4–6)
125 g (4½ oz) small new potatoes
125 g (4½ oz) shelled broad beans
50 g (2 oz) low-fat soft cream cheese
4 eggs
2 tbsp chopped thyme
freshly ground black pepper
2 tbsp olive oil
1 onion, peeled and roughly chopped
225 g (8 oz) courgettes, sliced
125 g (4½ oz) lightly cooked salmon, flaked
125 g (4½ oz) cooked, peeled prawns

1. Cook the potatoes and broad beans separately in boiling water until just tender; then drain thoroughly.

2. In a bowl, whisk together the cheese, eggs, thyme and pepper.

3. Heat the oil in a large, shallow, ovenproof pan. Add the onion, courgettes, potatoes and beans. Cook, stirring, for 2–3 minutes.

4. Add the salmon and prawns and pour in the egg mixture. As the eggs cook, push the mixture to the centre to allow the raw egg to flow down the edge of the pan.

Oaty Chestnut Flan

(Serves 8)

This unusual flan case is not only simple to make, but it can be made in advance and frozen.

Pastry

1 × 439 g (15½ oz) can chestnut purée
50 g (2 oz) polyunsaturated margarine
150 g (5 oz) porridge oats
2 tsp dried mixed herbs

Filling

225 g (8 oz) potato, peeled
225 g (8 oz) leeks
225 g (8 oz) parsnips, peeled
1 bouquet garni
1 red pepper, sliced
50 g (2 oz) polyunsaturated margarine
1 garlic clove, crushed
50 g (2 oz) cornflour
75 g (3 oz) Cheddar cheese
2 small courgettes, thinly sliced
30 ml (2 tbsp) chopped chives

1. In a bowl, cream the chestnut purée with the margarine until smooth; then stir in the porridge oats and herbs. Press the mixture into the base and sides of a 25 cm (10 in) round flan dish. Place in

a preheated oven at 180°C/350°F/Gas mark 4 and cook for 25–30 minutes or until crisp.

2. Meanwhile make the filling. Cut the potatoes, leeks and parsnips into chunks. Bring 600 ml (1 pint) water to the boil in a saucepan. Add the bouquet garni, potato, leeks, parsnips and red pepper. Cover and simmer for about 10 minutes or until the vegetables are all tender, drain in a colander; reserve the liquid and make up to 600 ml (1 pint) with water if necessary. Discard the bouquet garni.

3. Heat the margarine in a saucepan and fry the garlic for 1 minute. Off the heat, stir in the cornflour. Cook for 2 minutes, stirring. Gradually add the reserved liquid, then bring to the boil and simmer 2–3 minutes, stirring. Add the cheese, cooked vegetables, courgettes and chives and season to taste.

4. Spoon the vegetable mixture on to the flan case and serve at once.

Variation: Adapt this recipe by substituting vegetables that are in season.

Oaty Vegetable Crumble

(Serves 4)

Crumble
50 g (2 oz) polyunsaturated margarine
50 g (2 oz) rice flour
50 g (2 oz) porridge oats
50 g (2 oz) Cheddar cheese, grated
seasoning

Filling
1 onion, peeled
225 g (8 oz) carrots
225 g (8 oz) celery
50 g (2 oz) polyunsaturated margarine
30 ml (2 tbsp) plain flour
600 ml (1 pint) vegetable stock (home-made or low-sodium cube)

225 g (8 oz) French beans, halved
225 g (8 oz) courgettes sliced
30 ml (2 tbsp) chopped parsley
400 g (14 oz) can red kidney beans

1. Rub the margarine into the rice flour until it resembles fine bread-crumbs, stir in the oats, cheese and season to taste. Set aside while you make the filling.
2. Slice the onion, carrots and celery. Melt the margarine in a saucepan, add the onions and fry gently for 5 minutes until softened. Add the celery and carrots, cover and cook gently for 5 minutes.
3. Add the plain flour and cook gently, stirring for 1–2 minutes. Remove from the heat and gradually blend in the stock. Bring to the boil, stirring constantly; then simmer for 5 minutes. Season to taste.
4. Add the French beans and simmer for 5 minutes, then add the courgettes and parsley. Cook for a further 5 minutes or until the vegetables are just tender. Add the kidney beans to the vegeta-bles and heat through. Turn the mixture into a deep flameproof dish.
5. Pile the crumble mixture over the vegetables and bake at 190°C/375°F/Gas mark 5 for 35–40 minutes or until golden brown.

Vegetable and Dahl Jackets

(Serves 4)
30 ml (2 tbsp) vegetable oil
1 small onion, chopped
1 tbsp mild curry powder
75 g (3 oz) lentils
75 g (3 oz) French beans, trimmed and cut into 2.5 cm (1 in) lengths
50 g (2 oz) raisins
25 g (1 oz) desiccated coconut
200 ml (7 fl oz) vegetable stock
400 g (14 oz) canned, chopped tomatoes

4 hot baked potatoes
freshly ground black pepper
toasted, flaked coconut to garnish

1. Heat the oil and sauté the onion for 3 minutes, until soft.
2. Add the curry powder and lentils and cook for 5 minutes, stirring occasionally.
3. Add the beans, raisins, coconut, stock and tomatoes, cover and simmer for 20 minutes, stirring frequently.
4. Cut the tops off the potatoes and scoop out the centres. Cut the potato into chunks, add to the vegetable dahl and season with black pepper.
5. Spoon a little of the vegetable mixture into the potato skins and serve the remainder separately.
6. Garnish with a little toasted coconut.

DESSERTS – STAGE 1

Apple Custard

(Serves 4)
450 g (1 lb) eating apples, sliced
150 ml (5 fl oz) water
½ tsp ground cinnamon
2 eggs

1. Preheat the oven to 180°C/350°F/Gas mark 4.
2. Place the apples, water and cinnamon in a saucepan and cook gently until the apple softens and most of the water is absorbed.
3. Blend in a blender or food processor and allow to cool for 5–10 minutes.
4. Whisk the eggs and add a little at a time to the apple juice.
5. Pour the custard into a 20 cm (8 in) baking dish and bake for 25–30 minutes until browned on top and firm. Serve immediately.

Apple and Passion Fruit Delight

(Serves 4)

4 large eating apples (about 800 g/1¾ lb), chopped
¼ cup water
3 medium passion fruits
1 tablespoon concentrated apple juice
1 teaspoon grated orange rind
3 egg whites

1. Place the apple and water in a saucepan and bring to the boil. Cover, reduce the heat and simmer for 5 minutes or until the apples are tender.
2. Add the passion fruit, apple juice and orange rind and stir well, then leave to cool.
3. Beat the egg whites in a bowl until soft peaks form. Fold this into the apple mixture, and refrigerate for 1 hour before serving.

Baked Apples

(Serves 4)

4 cooking apples
4 dessertspoons of concentrated apple juice
4 cups of water
4 pinches of cinnamon

1. Wash and core the apples, and score around the centres in a circle, just breaking the skin.
2. Place the apples in an oven-proof dish.
3. Mix the concentrated apple juice with the water and the cinnamon.
4. Pour the apple juice over the apples.
5. Bake in a moderate oven 180°C/350°F/Gas mark 4 approximately 50–60 minutes.

Banana and Mixed Summer Berry Smoothie

(Serves 4)
4 medium bananas
225 g (8 oz) frozen summer berries (raspberries, strawberries,
redcurrants, blueberries)
600 ml (1 pint) ice-cold soya milk

1. Put all the ingredients into a blender or process with a hand
blender, pour into glasses and serve.

(**NB:** Frozen berries are better than fresh as they make a thicker, icier
consistency and very often they contain more nutrients.)

Banana and Tofu Cream

(Serves 4)
200 g (7 oz) firm tofu
200 g (7 oz) bananas, skinned
75 g (3 oz) ground almonds
1 pinch of cinnamon
2 tsp almond flakes

1. Blend or process the tofu and banana together. To obtain a creamy
texture, the mixture may need to be put through a sieve.
2. Add the ground almonds and mix well.
3. Spoon into 4 bowls and sprinkle with the cinnamon and a few
almond flakes.

Cranberry Sorbet

(Serves 4)
285 ml (½ pint) unsweetened orange juice
225 g (8 oz) fresh cranberries
285 ml (½ pint) water
2 egg whites
artificial sweetener to taste if necessary

1. Place the orange juice and cranberries in a saucepan together with the water. Bring to the boil. Cover the saucepan and simmer gently 2–3 minutes.
2. Strain the cranberries, keeping the cranberry juice in a separate bowl.
3. Blend the soft cranberries in a liquidiser and add the juices.
4. Allow to cool and add the sweetener, if necessary.
5. Put the cranberry mixture into a shallow dish and place in the freezer until semi-frozen.
6. Whisk the egg whites until stiff.
7. Remove the cranberry mixture from the freezer and break up the ice crystals that have formed.
8. Tip the semi-frozen sorbet into a bowl and fold in the whisked egg white.
9. Return the mixture to the container and freeze until firm.
10. When you are ready to serve, scoop the cranberry sorbet into decorative glasses.

Dried Fruit Compote

(Serves 4)

225 g (8 oz) mixture of dried fruits, eg peaches, prunes, apples, apricots and pears
150 ml (10 level tbsp) orange juice
4 whole cloves
4 × 2.5 cm (1 in) sticks cinnamon
juice and zest of 1 lemon
2 tbsp water (optional)

1. Wash the fruit and place it in a bowl with the orange juice, spices, lemon juice and zest.
2. Leave to soak overnight.
3. Next day, if the juice has been absorbed add 2 tablespoons of water. Then place the mixture in a saucepan, bring to the boil, cover and simmer on a very low heat for 10–15 minutes.
4. Transfer to a serving bowl, removing the cinnamon and cloves. Leave to cool or serve warm.

Fresh Fruit Salad

(Serves 4)

1 dessert apple, peeled and sliced
1 banana, peeled and sliced
4 tbsp (60 ml) lemon juice
1 orange, peeled and segmented
1 grapefruit, peeled and segmented
100 g (4 oz) seedless grapes
2 kiwi fruits, peeled and sliced
2 tbsp (30 ml) orange juice
4 sprigs of mint

1. Toss the apple and banana in the lemon juice. This will prevent discoloration.
2. Combine all fruits in a serving bowl, serve chilled and decorate with sprigs of mint.

Fruit Snow

(Serves 4)

400 g (14 oz) dessert apples, peeled, cored and thinly sliced
4 tbsp (30 ml) water
grated rind of ½ orange
1 large egg white, beaten until stiff
orange slices for garnish

1. Place apple, water and orange rind in a saucepan. Cover and cook gently, stirring occasionally until apples are soft.
2. Rub the apples through a sieve and let them cool.
3. Fold in the egg white and chill before serving. Serve with slices of orange to decorate.

Gooseberry Jelly

(Serves 6)
450 g (1 lb) gooseberries, topped and tailed
150 ml (½ pint) water
300 ml (½ pint) pure apple juice
concentrated apple juice to sweeten
4 tsp powdered gelatine
2 tbsp water
gooseberries to decorate

1. Very sparingly, oil a 1½ pint (30 fl oz/850 ml) jelly mould.
2. Simmer the gooseberries and water until soft.
3. Blend the fruit in a liquidiser.
4. Mix the purée with the apple juice, and a little extra concentrated apple juice to sweeten according to taste.
5. Mix the gelatine with 2 tablespoons of water in a small heat-proof bowl, place the bowl in hot water and stir until dissolved.
6. Add the gooseberry mixture to the gelatine mixture and mix thoroughly.
7. Pour into the prepared jelly mould and chill for 2–3 hours until set.
8. Turn the jelly carefully out on to a serving plate and decorate with gooseberries.

Jellied Grapefruit

(Serves 4)
2 large pink grapefruits, halved
300 ml (½ pint) unsweetened pineapple juice
150 ml (½ pint) unsweetened grapefruit juice
3 tsp gelatine

1. Scoop out the grapefruit segments from the grapefruit. Remove any pith from the segments and from the grapefruit shells.
2. Place the 4 grapefruit shells on a dish and divide the grapefruit segments evenly among them.

3. Mix together the fruit juices. Take 2 tablespoons of mixed juices and add to the gelatine. Place the bowl in hot water, and stir until the gelatine has dissolved.
4. Mix the gelatine solution with the remaining fruit juice mixture. Pour equal amounts into each grapefruit shell.
5. Place the shells in the fridge to set for 2–3 hours.

Peach Sundae

(Serves 4)
4 peaches
300 g (10 oz) raspberries
5 tsp sugar
2 tsp arrowroot
4 tsp shredded, or toasted, desiccated coconut

1. Skin the peaches by blanching them. (Pour boiling water over them, leave to cool briefly, and then place in cold water. The skins will then peel off easily.)
2. Halve the peaches and remove the stones.
3. Sieve the raspberries, making a purée.
4. Take a little of the raspberry purée and mix with the arrowroot into a paste.
5. Stir the arrowroot paste into the raspberry purée, and add the sugar.
6. Place the mixture in a saucepan and boil for 1 minute, stirring constantly.
7. When the mixture has cooled, pour the sauce over the peaches and sprinkle with the coconut.

Rhubarb and Ginger Mousse

(Serves 4)
455 g (1 lb) rhubarb
Juice and grated rind of ½
orange
3 tbsps clear honey
2 egg whites
2 tbsps (30ml) water
¼ tsps ground ginger
2 tsps powdered gelatine (Gelzone vegetarian alternative)

1. Trim the rhubarb and chop into 1 inch (2.5 cm) pieces.
2. Put the rhubarb into a pan with the honey, orange juice, rind and the ginger, and simmer gently until the fruit is soft.
3. Dissolve the gelatine in 2 tablespoons of water, placing the bowl in hot water. Stir until the gelatine is dissolved.
4. Add the gelatine mixture to the fruit and beat until smooth.
5. Cool the rhubarb mixture until it is half-set.
6. Whisk the egg whites until stiff and fold them lightly into the half set mixture.
7. Spoon into decorative glasses and chill until set.

Wheat-free Pastry

(Makes enough to line a 30-cm (12-in) flan dish)
100 g (4 oz) gluten-free flour (available from Doves Farm)
1 egg
50 g (2 oz) Pure margarine

1. Combine all the ingredients and form into a small ball.
2. Roll out on to greaseproof paper.
3. To keep pastry intact, place a flan dish face down on to the greaseproof paper and invert it. Lightly press the pastry down and around the sides of the flan dish. Fill and bake as directed, depending on which recipe is used for the filling.

DESSERTS – STAGE 2

Apple Charlotte

(Serves 4)

1 level tsp (5 ml) low-fat spread
450 g (1 lb) cooking apples
4 tbsp (60 ml) honey
75 g (3 oz) white breadcrumbs
4 tbsp (60 ml) already diluted apple juice
¼ level tsp (1.25 ml) ground ginger

1. Lightly grease 4 individual ovenproof dishes with low-fat spread.
2. Slice the apple and arrange half equally between the dishes.
3. Top with half the honey and sprinkle on half the breadcrumbs.
4. Repeat the layers until all the ingredients are used.
5. Pour over the apple juice and sprinkle on the ginger. Place in the oven at 180°C/350°F/Gas mark 4 for about 1 hour until the apples are tender and topping is crispy.

Berry Tofu Cream

(Serves 4)

200 g (7 oz) firm tofu
200 g (7 oz) mixed berries (strawberries, raspberries, blueberries)
75 g (3 oz) ground almonds
1 pinch of cinnamon
2 tsp flaked, toasted almonds

1. Blend or process the tofu and berries together. To obtain a creamy texture, the mixture may need to be put through a sieve or food mill.
2. Add the ground almonds and mix well.
3. Spoon into 4 bowls or glasses and sprinkle lightly with the cinnamon and a few almond flakes.

Variation: Substitute 200 g (7 oz) skinned bananas for the mixed berries.

Blackberries with Hazelnut Cheese

(Serves 4)
700 g (1½ lb) blackberries (fresh or frozen)
1 tbsp dark soft brown sugar
½ tbsp (7.5 ml) tropical fruit juice
55 g (2 oz) hazelnuts
1 tsp caster sugar
100 g (4 oz) cottage cheese

1. Clean and prepare the blackberries. Mix with the brown sugar and tropical fruit juice.
2. Toast the hazelnuts in a frying pan and add the caster sugar when the nuts are brown. Shake the pan continuously to coat the nuts in the melting sugar and set aside on a plate to cool.
3. Grind the caramel-coated nuts in a blender or coffee grinder and spread them out on a large sheet of greaseproof paper.
4. Divide the cottage cheese into 4 equal-sized balls, then roll them into the crushed nuts, gently pressing the nuts on to the surface of the cheese.
5. Place the individual cheeses on a plate and then into the refrigerator to set.
6. When you are about to serve, place the individual cheese balls in dessert glasses and surround each one with the berries.

Grapefruit Sorbet

(Serves 4)
2 grapefruit
425 ml (15 fl oz) water
about 3 tbsp concentrated apple juice
3 tbsp natural yogurt
2 egg whites
peeled grapefruit segments for decoration

1. Thinly pare the rind from the grapefruit and place the grapefruit rind and water into a pan. Simmer gently for 8 minutes and strain into a bowl.
2. Cut the fruit in half and squeeze out the juice.
3. Add the grapefruit juice to the liquid from the grapefruit rind and then add apple juice to taste.
4. Pour this liquid into a shallow freezer container and freeze until semi-frozen.
5. Turn the semi-frozen grapefruit mixture into a bowl and beat to break up the ice crystals.
6. Mix in the yogurt.
7. Whisk the egg whites until stiff and fold into the grapefruit and yogurt mixture gently.
8. Return to the freezer for 3 hours, or until firm.
9. Scoop out the sorbet into dessert glasses and decorate with peeled grapefruit segments.

Melon Ice Cream

(Serves 4)
1 medium melon (ogen or similar)
285 ml (½ pint) plain yogurt
concentrated apple juice to sweeten if necessary
16 raspberries to decorate

1. Halve the melon, scoop out the seeds and then scoop out the melon flesh and place in a liquidiser.
2. Liquidise the melon flesh and mix with the yogurt and concentrated apple juice as needed.
3. Place the melon and yogurt mixture in a shallow dish and freeze for 3 hours, or until firm.
4. Scoop the melon ice cream into dessert glasses and decorate with the raspberries.

Passion Fruit Fool

(Serves 4)

6 ripe passion fruit
140 ml (¼ pint) skimmed milk
3 tsp cornflour
2 tbsp (30 ml) water
140 ml (¼ pint) natural yogurt
1 tbsp (15 ml) clear honey

1. Halve the passion fruit and scoop the fruit pulp into a bowl.
2. Gently heat the skimmed milk.
3. Blend the cornflour and water into a smooth paste and then stir into the hot milk. Stir over the heat until the sauce has thickened, and remove to cool slightly.
4. Stir the yogurt and honey into the sauce and leave until cool.
5. Combine the sauce and the passion-fruit pulp and then spoon the mixture into serving dishes.
6. Chill for 3–4 minutes and serve from the refrigerator.

Tropical Crumble

(Serves 4)

4 bananas, sliced
2 tbsp brown sugar
2 tbsp pure maple syrup
50 g (2 oz) rice flour
50 g (2 oz) porridge oats
25 g (1 oz) soft brown sugar
15 g (1½ oz) desiccated coconut
50 g (2 oz) butter, melted

1. Place the sliced bananas, sugar and maple syrup in an ovenproof dish and cook under a low grill for 3 minutes.
2. Mix the dry ingredients together and pour over the melted butter.

3. Sprinkle this oaty topping over the bananas and grill under a moderate heat for 3 minutes, or until golden brown and crunchy.
4. Serve with custard or ice cream.

(**NB:** This topping works very well with any type of fresh fruit.)

Yogurt Ice Cream

(Serves 4)

225 g (8 oz) raspberries, plums, peaches or other soft fruit
1 tsp (5 ml) concentrated apple juice to sweeten
300 g (10 oz) natural yogurt
Mint sprig to decorate

1. Wash and prepare the fruit as necessary, and purée it in a liquidiser with the apple juice.
2. Place the mixture in the freezer for 2–3 hours until semi-frozen.
3. Remove the mixture from the freezer, add the yogurt and whisk well, then freeze until firm.
4. Place the yogurt ice cream in the refrigerator 30 minutes before serving to allow it to soften.
5. Scoop the ice cream into chilled dessert dishes and decorate with fruit or mint.

CAKES AND BISCUITS – STAGE 1

Gluten-free Scones

(Makes 6)

50 g (2 oz) rice flour
50 g (2 oz) buckwheat flour
100 g (4 oz) potato flour
(**Or** 200 g (8 oz) Dove's Farm gluten-free flour)
50 g (2 oz) ground almonds or soya flour
1 dessertspoon wheat-free baking powder
50 g (2 oz) butter or margarine
50 g (2 oz) caster sugar

150 ml (¼ pint) soya milk
1 egg, beaten

1. Combine the flours and baking powder in a large bowl.
2. Add the butter or margarine and mix with fingertips until it resembles fine breadcrumbs.
3. Stir in the sugar, soya milk and beaten egg and mix well.
4. The mixture will be fairly moist, so if you cannot roll it out, just place spoonfuls on to a baking tray. Brush the top with soya milk.
5. Bake at 200°C/425°F/Gas mark 7 for 10–15 minutes until golden brown.

Variations
Cheese scones (Stage 2 only)
Add 100 g (4 oz) grated Cheddar cheese
1 tsp mustard powder
1 dessertspoon mixed herbs

Fruit scones
Add 100 g (4 oz) mixed dried fruit

Sugar-free scones
Omit the sugar and serve with nut butters and sugar-free fruit spreads.

Nutty Fruit Tea Loaf

(Makes 8 slices)
375 g (12 oz) mixed dried fruit
juice and rind of 1 lemon
300 ml (½ pint) strong, hot Rooibosch tea
75 g (3 oz) whole almonds
75 g (3 oz) pecan nuts
300 g (10 oz) Doves Farm gluten-free flour
1 tsp ground mixed spice
1 tsp ground ginger
3 tsp wheat-free baking powder
1 egg, beaten
soya milk

1. Combine the dried fruit with the lemon juice and rind in a large bowl and leave to soak in the hot Rooibosch tea for at least 8 hours.
2. Toast the nuts until lightly golden and leave to cool.
3. Put the Doves Farm flour into a separate bowl with the spices and baking powder, then combine thoroughly with the toasted nuts, soaked fruit and remaining liquid. Add the egg and stir well. If the mixture appears too dry, add a few tablespoons of soya milk.
4. Line a 1 kg (2 lb) loaf tin, and put the tea loaf mixture in, roughly smoothing the top.
5. Bake at 150°C/300°F/Gas mark 2 approximately 1½–1¾ hours, or until well risen and firm to touch.
6. Serve cold, or lightly toasted with pure fruit jam or cheese.

Almond Macaroons

(Makes 18 biscuits)
2 large egg whites
150 g (6 oz) ground almonds
75 g (3 oz) unrefined caster sugar
18 almond halves

1. Put the unbeaten egg whites into a large bowl with the ground almonds, beat well, adding the caster sugar 1 tablespoon at a time.
2. Line biscuit trays with greaseproof paper.
3. Roll the mixture into balls and flatten with the palm of your hand.
4. Lay the flattened biscuits on to the trays and place an almond half in the middle of each biscuit.
5. Bake in a moderate oven at 180°C/350°F/Gas mark 4 for 25 minutes or until golden brown.

Banana Cake

(Makes 16 slices)

75 g (3 oz) dried dates
100 ml (4 fl oz) water
225 g (8 oz) banana, finely mashed
1 egg (size 3) whisked
75 g (3 oz) Doves Farm gluten-free flour
25 g (1 oz) soya flour
50 g (2 oz) ground almonds
1 tsp bicarbonate of soda
2.5 ml (½ tsp) vanilla essence
150 ml (5 fl oz) low-fat natural yogurt

1. Preheat the oven to 180°C/350°F/Gas mark 4.
2. Cook the dates in the water over a low heat until all the water has been absorbed. Blend in a food processor to a smooth paste.
3. Mix the cooled paste with the banana and egg, then fold in the flours, ground almonds and bicarbonate of soda. Stir in the vanilla essence and yogurt.
4. Lightly grease and flour a 20 cm (8 in) diameter baking tin and pour in the mixture.
5. Bake 35–40 minutes until the cake is brown on top and comes away from the tin.

Christmas Pudding

2 pint pudding basin
2 eggs
100 g (4 oz) Pure dairy-free margarine
100 g (4 oz) alternative breadcrumbs (wheat, oats, rye and barley free)
50 g (2 oz) brown rice flour
50 g (2 oz) cornflour
100 g (4 oz) molasses
1 large cooking apple, chopped
1 tsp cinnamon
1 tsp ginger

1 tsp mixed spice
200 g (8 oz) raisins
100 g (4 oz) sultanas
100 g (4 oz) currants
50 g (2 oz) mixed candied peel
1 grated carrot
50 g (2 oz) flaked almonds
zest of 1 large orange and 1 lemon
3 tbsp rum
3 tbsp brandy
3 tbsp port
1 tsp baking powder (wheat free)
½ tsp bicarbonate of soda
piece of muslin or cotton fabric
pressure cooker

1. Lightly grease the pudding basin.
2. Whisk the eggs and melt the margarine until soft.
3. Mix all the ingredients together and place in the pudding basin.
4. Cover with greaseproof paper and a layer of muslin or cotton. Tie with string and bring the sides of the muslin up and knot to make a handle, which will make it easier to lift out of the pressure cooker when cooked.
5. Pressure cook for 2 hours for or until cooked through.

Coconut Pyramids

(Makes 24)
4 egg yolks or 2 whole eggs
75 g (3 oz) unrefined caster sugar
juice and rind of half a lemon
250 g (8 oz) desiccated (dried and shredded) coconut

1. Beat the eggs and sugar until creamy.
2. Stir in the lemon juice, rind and coconut.

3. Form into pyramid shapes, either with your hands or using a moist egg cup, and place on a greased baking tray.
4. Bake at 190°C/375°F/Gas mark 5 20–25 minutes until the tips are golden brown.

Lemon and Almond Cake

175 g (6 oz) Pure dairy-free margarine
150 g (5 oz) unrefined caster sugar
3 eggs
175 g (6 oz) Doves Farm gluten-free flour
50 g (2 oz) ground almonds
grated rind and juice of 1 lemon
½ tsp almond essence

To finish
2 lemons
2 tbsp clear honey

1. Preheat the oven to 160°/325°F/Gas mark 3. Grease and line a 20 cm (8 in) loose-bottomed round cake tin.
2. Place all the cake ingredients in a large bowl and mix well. Beat with a wooden spoon or electric whisk for 2–3 minutes until light and fluffy.
3. Turn mixture into the cake tin and smooth the top. Pare the rind and pith of the two lemons, then slice into thin round slices and place on top of the cake.
4. Bake 50–60 minutes until golden and firm. Cool in tin for 10 minutes, then release the sides and cool on a wire rack. Warm the honey, brush over the cake and serve.

CAKES AND BISCUITS – STAGE 2

Crunchy Seed Squares

(Makes 8 slices)

3 tbsp brown rice syrup
1 tbsp honey
7 tbsp walnut oil
75 g (3 oz) porridge oats
75 g (3 oz) soya flour
2 tbsp ground almonds
1 tbsp sunflower seeds
1 tbsp pumpkin seeds
1 tbsp linseeds
50 g (2 oz) flaked almonds

1. Warm the brown rice syrup, honey and walnut oil and mix thoroughly with the dry ingredients.
2. Press into a greased 23 cm × 23 cm (9 in × 9 in) square cake tin and bake in a preheated oven at 180°C/350°F/Gas mark 4 for 25 minutes.

Note: Use buckwheat flakes or Doves Farm gluten-free flour for a totally wheat and gluten-free version. You may need to add a little more syrup and oil if the mixture appears too dry.

Nutritional content of food

In order to make your diet more nutrient dense, go through these lists and select the foods from each nutrient that you enjoy and include them in your regime at the appropriate stage. Remember that dairy products, wheat, oats, barley and rye are only allowed in Stage 2.

Unless stated otherwise, foods listed are raw.

Vitamin A – Retinol
Micrograms per 100 g (3.5 oz)

Skimmed milk	1
Semi-skimmed milk	21
Grilled herring	49
Whole milk	52
Porridge made with milk	56
Cheddar cheese	325
Margarine	800
Butter	815
Lamb's liver	15,000

Vitamin B1 – Thiamin
Milligrams per 100 g (3.5 oz)

Peaches	0.02
Cottage cheese	0.02
Cox's apple	0.03
Full-fat milk	0.04
Skimmed milk	0.04
Semi-skimmed milk	0.04
Cheddar cheese	0.04
Bananas	0.04
White grapes	0.04
French beans	0.04
Low-fat yogurt	0.05
Cantaloupe melon	0.05
Tomato	0.06
Green peppers, raw	0.07
Boiled egg	0.08
Roast chicken	0.08
Grilled cod	0.08
Haddock, steamed	0.08
Roast turkey	0.09
Mackerel, cooked	0.09
Savoy cabbage, boiled	0.10
Oranges	0.10
Brussels sprouts	0.10
Potatoes, new, boiled	0.11
Soya beans, boiled	0.12
Red peppers, raw	0.12
Lentils, boiled	0.14
Steamed salmon	0.20
Corn	0.20
White spaghetti, boiled	0.21
Almonds	0.24
White self-raising flour	0.30
Plaice, steamed	0.30
Bacon, cooked	0.35
Walnuts	0.40

Wholemeal flour	0.47
Lamb's kidney	0.49
Brazil nuts	1.00
Corn flakes	1.00
Rice Krispies	1.00
Wheatgerm	2.01

Vitamin B2 – Riboflavin
Milligrams per 100 g (3.5 oz)

Cabbage, boiled	0.01
Potatoes, boiled	0.01
Brown rice, boiled	0.02
Pear	0.03
Wholemeal spaghetti, boiled	0.03
White self-raising flour	0.03
Orange	0.04
Spinach, boiled in salted water	0.05
Baked beans	0.06
Banana	0.06
White bread	0.06
Green peppers, raw	0.08
Lentils, boiled	0.08
Hovis	0.09
Soya beans, boiled	0.09
Wholemeal bread	0.09
Wholemeal flour	0.09
Peanuts	0.10
Baked salmon	0.11
Red peppers, raw	0.15
Full-fat milk	0.17
Avocado	0.18
Grilled herring	0.18
Semi-skimmed milk	0.18
Roast chicken	0.19
Roast turkey	0.21

Cottage cheese	0.26
Soya flour	0.31
Boiled prawns	0.34
Boiled egg	0.35
Topside of beef, cooked	0.35
Leg of lamb, cooked	0.38
Cheddar cheese	0.40
Muesli	0.70
Almonds	0.75
Corn flakes	1.50
Rice Krispies	1.50

Vitamin B3 – Niacin
Milligrams per 100 g (3.5 oz)

Boiled egg	0.07
Cheddar cheese	0.07
Full-fat milk	0.08
Skimmed milk	0.09
Semi-skimmed milk	0.09
Cottage cheese	0.13
Cox's apple	0.20
Cabbage, boiled	0.30
Orange	0.40
Baked beans	0.50
Potatoes, boiled	0.50
Soya beans, boiled	0.50
Lentils, boiled	0.60
Banana	0.70
Tomato	1.00
Avocado	1.10
Green peppers, raw	1.10
Brown rice	1.30
Wholemeal spaghetti, boiled	1.30
White self-raising flour	1.50
Grilled cod	1.70
White bread	1.70

Soya flour	2.00		Baked beans	0.12
Red peppers, raw	2.20		Boiled egg	0.12
Almonds	3.10		Red kidney beans, cooked	0.12
Grilled herring	4.00		Wholemeal bread	0.12
Wholemeal bread	4.10		Tomatoes	0.14
Hovis	4.20		Almonds	0.15
Wholemeal flour	5.70		Cauliflower	0.15
Muesli	6.50		Brussels sprouts	0.19
Topside of beef, cooked	6.50		Sweetcorn, boiled	0.21
Leg of lamb, cooked	6.60		Leg of lamb, cooked	0.22
Baked salmon	7.00		Grapefruit juice	0.23
Roast chicken	8.20		Roast chicken	0.26
Roast turkey	8.50		Lentils, boiled	0.28
Boiled prawns	9.50		Banana	0.29
Peanuts	13.80		Brazil nuts	0.31
Corn flakes	16.00		Potatoes, boiled	0.32
Rice Krispies	16.00		Roast turkey	0.33
			Grilled herring	0.33

Vitamin B6 – Pyridoxine

Milligrams per 100 g (3.5 oz)

			Topside of beef, cooked	0.33
Carrots	0.05		Avocado	0.36
Full-fat milk	0.06		Grilled cod	0.38
Skimmed milk	0.06		Baked salmon	0.57
Semi-skimmed milk	0.06		Soya flour	0.57
Satsuma	0.07		Hazelnuts	0.59
White bread	0.07		Peanuts	0.59
White rice	0.07		Walnuts	0.67
Cabbage, boiled	0.08		Muesli	1.60
Cottage cheese	0.08		Corn flakes	1.80
Cox's apple	0.08		Rice Krispies	1.80
Wholemeal pasta	0.08		Special K	2.20
Frozen peas	0.09			
Spinach, boiled	0.09			
Cheddar cheese	0.10			

Vitamin B12 – Cyanocobalamine

Micrograms per 100 g (3.5 oz)

Orange	0.10		Tempeh	0.10
Broccoli	0.11		Miso	0.20
Hovis	0.11		Quorn	0.30

Full-fat mik	0.40	Tuna in oil	5.00
Skimmed milk	0.40	Herring, cooked	6.00
Semi-skimmed milk	0.40	Herring roe, fried	6.00
Marmite	0.50	Steamed salmon	6.00
Cottage cheese	0.70	Bovril	8.30
Choux buns	1.00	Mackerel, fried	10.00
Eggs, boiled	1.00	Rabbit, stewed	10.00
Eggs, poached	1.00	Cod's roe, fried	11.00
Halibut, steamed	1.00	Pilchards canned in	
Lobster, boiled	1.00	tomato juice	12.00
Sponge cake	1.00	Oysters, raw	15.00
Turkey, white meat	1.00	Nori seaweed	27.50
Waffles	1.00	Sardines in oil	28.00
Cheddar cheese	1.20	Lamb's kidney, fried	79.00
Eggs, scrambled	1.20		
Squid	1.30		

Folate/Folic Acid

Micrograms per 100 g (3.5 oz)

Eggs, fried	1.60	Cox's apple	4.00
Shrimps, boiled	1.80	Leg of lamb, cooked	4.00
Parmesan cheese	1.90	Full-fat milk	6.00
Beef, lean	2.00	Skimmed milk	6.00
Cod, baked	2.00	Semi-skimmed milk	6.00
Corn flakes	2.00	Porridge with semi-skimmed	
Pork, cooked	2.00	milk	7.00
Raw beef mince	2.00	Turnip, baked	8.00
Rice Krispies	2.00	Sweet potato, boiled	8.00
Steak, lean, grilled	2.00	Cucumber	9.00
Edam cheese	2.10	Grilled herring	10.00
Eggs, whole, battery	2.40	Roast chicken	10.00
Milk, dried, whole	2.40	Avocado	11.00
Milk, dried, skimmed	2.60	Grilled cod	12.00
Eggs, whole, free-range	2.70	Banana	14.00
Kambu seaweed	2.80	Roast turkey	15.00
Squid, frozen	2.90	Carrots	17.00
Taramasalata	2.90	Sweet potato	17.00
Duck, cooked	3.00	Tomatoes	17.00
Turkey, dark meat	3.00	Topside of beef, cooked	17.00
Grapenuts	5.00		

Swede, boiled	18.00	Artichoke	68.00
Strawberries	20.00	Hazelnuts	72.00
Brazil nuts	21.00	Spinach, boiled	90.00
Red peppers, raw	21.00	Brussels sprouts	110.00
Green peppers, raw	23.00	Peanuts	110.00
Rye bread	24.00	Muesli	140.00
Dates, fresh	25.00	Sweetcorn, boiled	150.00
New potatoes, boiled	25.00	Asparagus	155.00
Grapefruit	26.00	Chickpeas	180.00
Oatcakes	26.00	Lamb's liver, fried	240.00
Cottage cheese	27.00	Corn flakes	250.00
Baked salmon	29.00	Rice Krispies	250.00
Cabbage, boiled	29.00	Calf's liver, fried	320.00
Onions, boiled	29.00		
White bread	29.00		

Vitamin C

Milligrams per 100 g (3.5 oz)

Orange	31.00	Full-fat milk	1.00
Baked beans	33.00	Skimmed milk	1.00
Cheddar cheese	33.00	Semi-skimmed milk	1.00
Clementines	33.00	Red kidney beans	1.00
Raspberries	33.00	Carrots	2.00
Satsuma	33.00	Cucumber	2.00
Blackberries	34.00	Muesli with dried fruit	2.00
Rye crispbread	35.00	Apricots, raw	6.00
Potato, baked in skin	36.00	Avocado	6.00
Radish	38.00	Pear	6.00
Boiled egg	39.00	Potato, boiled	6.00
Hovis	39.00	Spinach, boiled	8.00
Wholemeal bread	39.00	Cox's apple	9.00
Red kidney beans, boiled	42.00	Turnip	10.00
Potato, baked	44.00	Banana	11.00
Frozen peas	47.00	Frozen peas	12.00
Almonds	48.00	Lamb's liver, fried	12.00
Parsnips, boiled	48.00	Pineapple	12.00
Cauliflower	51.00	Dried skimmed milk	13.00
Green beans, boiled	57.00	Gooseberries	14.00
Broccoli	64.00	Raw dates	14.00
Walnuts	66.00		

Melon	17.00	Cucumber	0.07
Tomatoes	17.00	Cottage cheese	0.08
Cabbage, boiled	20.00	Full-fat milk	0.09
Canteloupe melon	26.00	Cabbage, boiled	0.10
Cauliflower	27.00	Leg of lamb, cooked	0.10
Satsuma	27.00	Cauliflower	0.11
Peach	31.00	Roast chicken	0.11
Raspberries	32.00	Frozen peas	0.18
Bran flakes	35.00	Red kidney beans, cooked	0.20
Grapefruit	36.00	Wholemeal bread	0.20
Mangoes	37.00	Orange	0.24
Nectarine	37.00	Topside of beef, cooked	0.26
Kumquats	39.00	Banana	0.27
Broccoli	44.00	Brown rice, boiled	0.30
Lychees	45.00	Grilled herring	0.30
Unsweetened apple juice	49.00	Lamb's liver, fried	0.32
Orange	54.00	Baked beans	0.36
Kiwi fruit	59.00	Cornflakes	0.40
Brussels sprouts	60.00	Pear	0.50
Strawberries	77.00	Cheddar cheese	0.53
Blackcurrants	115.00	Carrots	0.56
		Lettuce	0.57

Vitamin D

Micrograms per 100 g (3.5 oz)

		Cox's apple	0.59
Skimmed milk	0.01	Grilled cod	0.59
Whole milk	0.03	Rice Krispies	0.60
Fromage frais	0.05	Plums	0.61
Cheddar cheese	0.26	Unsweetened orange	
Corn flakes	2.80	juice	0.68
Rice Krispies	2.80	Leeks	0.78
Kellogg's Start	4.20	Sweetcorn, boiled	0.88
Margarine	8.00	Brussels sprouts	0.90
		Broccoli	1.10
		Boiled egg	1.11

Vitamin E

Milligrams per 100 g (3.5 oz)

		Tomato	1.22
		Watercress	1.46
Semi-skimmed milk	0.03	Parsley	1.70
Boiled potatoes	0.06	Spinach, boiled	1.71

Olives	1.99	White rice, boiled	18.00
Butter	2.00	Grilled cod	22.00
Onions, dried raw	2.69	Lentils, boiled	22.00
Mushrooms, fried in		Baked salmon	29.00
corn oil	2.84	Green peppers, raw	30.00
Avocado	3.20	Young carrots	30.00
Muesli	3.20	Grilled herring	33.00
Walnuts	3.85	Wholemeal flour	38.00
Peanut butter	4.99	Turnips, baked	45.00
Olive oil	5.10	Orange	47.00
Sweet potato, baked	5.96	Baked beans	48.00
Brazil nuts	7.18	Wholemeal bread	54.00
Peanuts	10.09	Boiled egg	57.00
Pine nuts	13.65	Peanuts	60.00
Rapeseed oil	18.40	Cottage cheese	73.00
Almonds	23.96	Soya beans, boiled	83.00
Hazelnuts	24.98	White bread	100.00
Sunflower oil	48.70	Full-fat milk	115.00
		Hovis	120.00

Calcium

Milligrams per 100 g (3.5 oz)

		Muesli	120.00
Cox's apple	4.00	Skimmed milk	120.00
Brown rice, boiled	4.00	Semi-skimmed milk	120.00
Potatoes, boiled	5.00	Prawns, boiled	150.00
Banana	6.00	Spinach, boiled	150.00
Topside of beef, cooked	6.00	Brazil nuts	170.00
White pasta, boiled	7.00	Yogurt, low-fat, plain	190.00
Tomato	7.00	Soya flour	210.00
White spaghetti, boiled	7.00	Almonds	240.00
Leg of lamb, cooked	8.00	White self-raising flour	450.00
Red peppers, raw	8.00	Sardines	550.00
Roast chicken	9.00	Sprats, fried	710.00
Roast turkey	9.00	Cheddar cheese	720.00
Avocado	11.00	Whitebait, fried	860.00
Pear	11.00		

Chromium

Micrograms per 100 g (3.5 oz)

Butter	15.00
Corn flakes	15.00
Egg yolk	183.00

Molasses	121.00
Brewer's yeast	117.00
Beef	57.00
Hard cheese	56.00
Liver	55.00
Fruit juices	47.00
Wholemeal bread	42.00

Iron
Milligrams per 100 g (3.5 oz)

Semi-skimmed milk	0.05
Skimmed milk	0.06
Full-fat milk	0.06
Cottage cheese	0.10
Orange	0.10
Cox's apple	0.20
Pear	0.20
White rice	0.20
Banana	0.30
Cabbage, boiled	0.30
Cheddar cheese	0.30
Avocado	0.40
Grilled cod	0.40
Potatoes, boiled	0.40
Young carrots, boiled	0.40
Brown rice, boiled	0.50
Tomato	0.50
White pasta, boiled	0.50
Baked salmon	0.80
Roast chicken	0.80
Roast turkey	0.90
Grilled herring	1.00
Red peppers, raw	1.00
Boiled prawns	1.10
Green peppers, raw	1.20
Baked beans	1.40

Wholemeal spaghetti, boiled	1.40
White bread	1.60
Spinach, boiled	1.70
Boiled egg	1.90
White self-raising four	2.00
Brazil nuts	2.50
Peanuts	2.50
Leg of lamb, cooked	2.70
Wholemeal bread	2.70
Topside of beef, cooked	2.80
Almonds	3.00
Soya beans, boiled	3.00
Lentils, boiled	3.50
Hovis	3.70
Wholemeal flour	3.90
Muesli	5.60
Corn flakes	6.70
Rice Krispies	6.70
Soya flour	6.90

Magnesium
Milligrams per 100 g (3.5 oz)

Butter	2.00
Cox's apple	6.00
Turnip, baked	6.00
Young carrots	6.00
Tomato	7.00
Cottage cheese	9.00
Orange	10.00
Full-fat milk	11.00
White rice, boiled	11.00
Semi-skimmed milk	11.00
Skimmed milk	12.00
Boiled egg	12.00
Corn flakes	14.00
Potatoes, boiled	14.00

Red peppers, raw	14.00
White pasta, boiled	15.00
Wholemeal spaghetti, boiled	15.00
White self-raising flour	20.00
Green peppers, raw	24.00
Roast chicken	24.00
Topside of beef, cooked	24.00
White bread	24.00
Avocado	25.00
Cheddar cheese	25.00
Grilled cod	26.00
Roast turkey	27.00
Leg of lamb, cooked	28.00
Baked salmon	29.00
Baked beans	31.00
Spinach, boiled	31.00
Grilled herring	32.00
Banana	34.00
Lentils, boiled	34.00
Boiled prawns	42.00
Wholemeal spaghetti, boiled	42.00
Brown rice, boiled	43.00
Hovis	56.00
Soya beans, boiled	63.00
Wholemeal bread	76.00
Muesli	85.00
Wholemeal flour	120.00
Peanuts	210.00
Soya flour	240.00
Almonds	270.00
Brazil nuts	410.00

Selenium
Micrograms per 100 g (3.5 oz)

Full-fat milk	1.00
Semi-skimmed milk	1.00
Skimmed milk	1.00
Baked beans	2.00
Corn flakes	2.00
Orange	2.00
Peanuts	3.00
Almonds	4.00
Cottage cheese	4.00
White rice	4.00
White self-raising flour	4.00
Soya beans, boiled	5.00
Boiled egg	11.00
Cheddar cheese	12.00
White bread	28.00
Wholemeal bread	35.00
Lentils, boiled	40.00
Wholemeal flour	53.00

Zinc
Milligrams per 100 g (3.5 oz)

Butter	0.10
Pear	0.10
Orange	0.10
Red peppers, raw	0.10
Banana	0.20
Young carrots	0.20
Corn flakes	0.30
Potatoes, boiled	0.30
Avocado	0.40
Full-fat milk	0.40
Skimmed milk	0.40
Green peppers, raw	0.40
Semi-skimmed milk	0.40
Baked beans	0.50
Grilled cod	0.50
Grilled herring	0.50

White pasta	0.50
Tomatoes	0.50
Cottage cheese	0.60
Spinach, boiled	0.60
White bread	0.60
White self-raising flour	0.60
Brown rice	0.70
White rice	0.70
Soya beans, boiled	0.90
Wholemeal spaghetti, boiled	1.10
Boiled egg	1.30
Lentils, boiled	1.40
Roast chicken	1.50
Boiled prawns	1.60
Wholemeal bread	1.80
Hovis	2.10
Cheddar cheese	2.30
Roast turkey	2.40
Muesli	2.50
Wholemeal flour	2.90
Almonds	3.20
Peanuts	3.50
Brazil nuts	4.20
Leg of lamb, cooked	5.30
Topside of beef, cooked	5.50

Essential Fatty Acids

Exact amounts of these fats are hard to quantify. Good sources for the two families of essential fatty acids are given.

Omega-6 Series Essential Fatty Acids

Sunflower oil
Rapeseed oil
Corn oil
Almonds
Walnuts
Brazil nuts
Sunflower seeds
Soya products including tofu

Omega-3 Series Essential Fatty Acids

Mackerel ⎫
Herring ⎬ fresh cooked or smoked/pickled
Salmon ⎭

Walnuts and walnut oil
Rapeseed oil
Soya products and soy bean oil

Weekly diary and review

	SCORE	
	Before	*After*
Is my diet good for me?	_____	_____
Am I in good nutritional shape?	_____	_____
Food sensitivity test	_____	_____
Food craving test	_____	_____
Caffeine test	_____	_____
Alcohol test	_____	_____
Tobacco test	_____	_____
Do I love myself?	_____	_____
How stressed am I?	_____	_____
How's my libido?	_____	_____
Total Score	_____	_____

Deduct your after score from your before

score to get your Personal Balance Score (PBS)   _____

Possible nutritional deficiencies

_____

_____

_____

_____

Special dietary recommendations

_____

_____

_____

_____

Supplements I need to take

_____

_____

_____

_____

My fitness score _____

Initial fitness score _____

Fitness category

Very unfit ☐   Moderately unfit ☐   Not as fit as I should be ☐   Moderately fit ☐

Fit ☐   In excellent physical condition ☐

My exercise plan

_____

_____

_____

_____

My relaxation plan

_____

_____

_____

_____

Lifestyle changes I need to make

_____

_____

_____

_____

Weekly Diary

Date:

Please complete the diary on a daily basis and grade symptoms on a scale of 0–3 according to severity with:

0 = None, 1 = Mild, 2 = Moderate, 3 = Severe

	Breakfast	Lunch	Dinner	Snacks	Exercise	Supplements	Relaxation	Symptoms	Reactions
Day 1									
Day 2									
Day 3									
Day 4									
Day 5									
Day 6									
Day 7									

Review

White list = Foods and drinks that you seem well on
Grey list = Foods and drinks that you are currently unsure of
Black list = Foods and drinks you had a reaction to

Stage 1	White list	Grey list	Black list

Stage 2	White list	Grey list	Black list

Stage 3	White list	Grey list	Black list

Healthy shopping options

Cakes and biscuits

Bakers Delight Gluten Free
Bramley Apple Tarts
Cake Bars
Maple and Pecan Fruit Cake
Sponge Puddings

The Village Bakery Organic and Gluten Free
4 Fruit Organic Bar
4 Nut Organic Bar
4 Seed Organic Bar
Apricot Slice
Blue Cheese Biscuits
Borrowdale Teabread
Butter Flapjack
Carrot Cake
Celebration Fruit Cake
Chocolate Almond Cake
Chocolate and Orange Brownies
Date Slice
Farmhouse Cake
Fruit Cake
Fruit, Nut and Seed Bar
Ginger Biscuits
Ginger Cake
Hazelnutter
Lemon Cake
Oatcakes
Orange and Vanilla Cake
Rich Fruit Cake
Savoury Biscuits
Savoury Seed Biscuits

Organic Gluten-free Christmas Range
Christmas Cake
Christmas Pudding
Fairtrade Christmas Cake
Mince Pies

Nairn's Wheat Free
Cheese Oat Cakes
Fine Milled Oat Cakes
Fruit and Spice Wheat Free Biscuits
Mini Oat Cakes
Mixed Berries Wheat Free Biscuits
Rough Oat Cakes
Savoury Biscuit Collection
Stem Ginger Wheat Free Biscuits
Wheat Free Biscuits

Orgran Fruit
Filled Blueberry Bar

Bread

Bakers Delight
Gluten, Wheat and Dairy Free Bread

Sunnyvale
Flax Corn Rice Sourdough
Gluten Free Mixed Grain Sourdough Bread

The Village Bakery
Baltic Rye Bread (rye and wheat bread with molasses and caraway
    made to a Latvian recipe)
Borodinsky (Russian rye bread flavoured with malt and coriander)
Brazil Nut and Apricot Bread
Brazil Nut and Linseed Bread
Campagne (French country bread made with natural leaven)
Gluten Free Bread (made with maize flour, chestnut flour, lupin flour
    and linseeds)
Hadrian (hand worked, naturally leavened spelt bread with raisin
    juice, inspired by the Romans)
Pane Toscano (naturally leavened, unsalted bread made in the Tuscan
    tradition)

Raisin Borodinsky (moist fruit loaf – malted rye and organic raisins)

Rossisky (Russian inspired rye bread based on a sourdough from Kostroma on the Volga River)

Sunflower Bread (wholemeal bread with sunflower seeds in the crumb and baked into the crust)

Ten Seed Bread (ten different types of seeds in the crumb and on the crust)

Wholemeal (made with a ripened dough)

Burgen
Cholesterol Loaf
Hi Bran Loaf
Soya and Linseed Loaf

Vogel
Breads.

Coffee substitutes

Bambu
Barleycup Granules
Barleycup Organic (instant cereal drink)
Organic Instant Coffee Substitute (from organically grown chicory, figs, cereals and acorns)

Cotswold
Dandelion Coffee (roasted dandelion root coffee)

Foods containing soya

Drinks
So Good soya milk essential
So Good soya low fat drink
Alpro plain fresh milk
Alpro milk with added calcium and vitamins
Alpro vanilla flavoured milk
Provamel chocolate soya drink

Spreads and breads
Waitrose pure organic soya butter spread
Waitrose sunflower spread

Holland & Barrett pure soya spread
Cauldron Aromatic herb and soya bean pate
Spreadable soya and mushroom pate
Burgen bread with soya and linseed
Vogel brown soya bread
Cauldron soya and mushroom pate
Cauldron tomato, lentil and basil pate
Cauldron roasted vegetable and feta pate

Cheese substitutes
Toffiti creamy smooth herbs and chives, cream cheese style
Toffiti cream cheese style with garlic and herbs
Toffiti cream cheese style, orginal
Toffiti mozzarella-style slices

Instead of meat and fish
Cauldron beech smoked tofu
Cauldron Lincolnshire veggie sausages
Cauldron carrot, peanut & onion burgers
Vegideli sage & marjoram sausages
Holland & Barrett porkless pies
Holland & Barrett Scotch eggs
Granovita vegetable frankfurters
Vegideli fish style fingers
Fudco soya chunks
Fudco soya mince

Desserts
Alpro cherry peach and mango yoghurts
Alpro Oy soya yoghurt
Alpro Fruits of the forest with added calcium
Alpro Custard with added calcium
Organic chocolate custard
Alpro cream alternative
Tofutti organic chocolate soya dessert
Tofutti organic mango/passion fruit soya dessert
Organic apple and cinnamon pancake mix
Granovita soyage cherry dessert

Cereals and nuts
Food Doctor roasted nuts
CanMar golden roasted milled flax seed with real blueberries

CanMar golden roasted milled flax seed with real apples
CanMar golden roasted milled flax seed, ready to eat
CanMar whole roasted flax seeds
Natural Harvest soya bran
Vogel soya and linseed cereal
Nature's Path organic power cereal with flaxseed, soy, blueberry

Cooking
Nature's Harvest soya flour
Community Foods soya flour
Neal's Yard organic soya beans
Nature's Harvest natural soya chunks
Nature's Harvest savoury soya chunks
Nature's Harvest natural mince
Nature's Harvest savoury soya mince
Birds Eye tinned soya beans

Sauces and Dressings

Meridian Free From Dairy, Wheat and Gluten
Creamy White Wine and Mushroom Sauce
Dark Tahini
Garlic and Herb Dip
Green Pesto
Hoot Salsa
Korma Sauce
Light Tahini
Organic Brown Sauce
Organic Cool Salsa Tomato Dip
Organic Cranberry Sauce – seasonal only
Organic Dark Tahini
Organic French Dressing
Organic Hot Salsa Tomato Dip
Organic Light Tahini
Organic Mayonnaise
Organic Salad Cream
Organic Sweet Pickle
Organic Tomato and Apple Chutney
Organic Tomato Ketchup
Red Pesto

Salad Cream
Shovu Soya Sauce
Sun Dried Tomato Sauce
Tamari Soya Sauce
Teriyaki Soya Sauce
Tikka Masala Sauce
Tomato Ketchup
Yeast Extract
Yeast Extract, Reduced Salt

Meridian Pasta Sauces
Organic Mushroom Pasta Sauce
Organic Red Pepper and Sweet Chilli Pasta Sauce
Organic Spanish Olive Pasta Sauce

Doves Farm
Apple and Sultana Flapjack
BioBiz
Cornflakes
Easy (a corn flake cereal bar with dried fruits and nuts)
Lemon Zest Cookies (zesty crystallised lemon pieces baked into a
    lemon cookie)
Raisin Honeys (wholemeal cookie)
Tasty (rice pops and chocolate blended into a chewy, crunchy, crispy
    chocolate breakfast bar)
Traditional Butter Flapjack

Swedish Glace non-dairy soft scoop frozen dessert
Caramel
Mocha and Coffee Ripple
Raspberry
Vanilla

Glutano gluten free foods
Brown Rice Fettuccini
Brown Rice Macaroni
Macaroni
Pasta Spirals
Rice Pasta Lasagne
Spagghetti
Tagliatelle
Tri Colour Pasta

Pure Products for gluten and wheat free baking
Gluten Free Blended Flou
Potato Starch Flour
Rice Flour
Tapioca Flour

Spreads (from Meridian, Whole Earth and St Dalfours)

100 per cent all fruit taste
Apricot Spread
Blackcurrant Spread
Grapefruit Spread
Morello Cherry Spread
Organic Apricot Spread
Organic Blackcurrant Spread
Organic Breakfast Spread Seville Orange
Organic Cherries and Berries Spread
Organic Cranberry and Orange Spread
Organic Morello Cherry Spread
Organic Raspberry Spread
Organic Strawberry Spread
Organic Wild Blueberry Spread
Pineapple and Ginger Spread
Raspberry Spread
Seville Orange Spread
Strawberry Spread
Tropical Fruit Spread
Wild Blueberry Spread

Nut butters (from Meridian, Whole Earth and St Dalfours)

100 per cent pure nut butter
Almond Butter
Brazil Nut Butter
Cashew Butter
Hazel Butter
Organic Peanut Butter, Crunchy
Organic Peanut Butter, Crunchy, No Salt
Peanut Butter, Crunchy

Peanut Butter, Smooth
Peanut Butter, Smooth, No Salt
Walnut Butter

Fruit juices

100 per cent pure juice
Apple and Blackcurrant Juice Concentrate
Apple Juice Concentrate
Organic Apple Juice Concentrate
Pear Juice Concentrate

Syrups

Barley Malt Extract
Date Syrup
Organic Blackstrap Molasses
Organic Maple Syrup

Tins

Orgran
Tinned Spaghetti (Stonemilled rice/yellow split pea spaghetti)

You can order direct from the following websites:

www.glutenfreefoodsdirect.co.uk
www.wheatanddairyfree.com
www.village-bakery.com
www.moilas.co.uk
www.dovesfarm.co.uk

Recommended reading and further information

Books:

Ackland, Lesley, *15 Minute Pilates*, HarperCollins, 1998.

Black, Jack, *Mindstore: The Ultimate Mental Fitness Programme*, HarperCollins, 1995.

Buzan, Tony, *Use Your Head*, BBC Books, 2003.

Cappacchione, Lucia, *Recovery of Your Inner Child*, Simon & Schuster, New York, 1991.

— *Visioning*, Jeremy P Tarcher, 2000.

Carr, Allen, *The Only Way to Stop Smoking Permanently*, Penguin Books Ltd, 1995.

Devereux, Godfrey, *15-Minute Yoga*, HarperCollins, 2000.

Donkersloot, Mary and Hyder-Ferry, Linda, *The How to Stop Smoking and Not Gain Weight Cookbook*, Three Rivers Press, 1999.

Greenspan, Miriam, *Healing through the Dark Emotions*, Shambhala Publications, 2004.

Harrold, Fiona, *The 10-Minute Life Coach*, Hodder & Stoughton Ltd, 2003.

Jennings, Tony and Philips, Georges, *My Little Book of NLP, Neuro Linguistic Programming*, ICET Paperback, 2000.

Kehoe, John, *Mind Power into the 21st Century*, Zoetic Inc, 1997.

McGraw, Dr Phil, *Life Strategies*, Hyperion, New York, 1999.

— *Life Strategies Workbook*, Hyperion, New York, 2000.

— *Relationship Rescue*, Hyperion, New York, 2000.

McKenna, Paul, *Change your Life in 7 Days*, Bantam Press, 2003.

— *How to Mend Your Broken Heart*, Bantam Press, 2003.

Riley, Gillian, *How to Stop Smoking and Stay Stopped For Good*, Vermilion, 2003.

Shakti, Gawain, *Creative Visualisation*, New World Library, 2002.

Stewart, Dr Alan and Maryon, *The Natural Health Bible*, Vermilion, 2001.

— *No More PMS*, Vermilion, 1997.

Stewart, Maryon, *Cruising through the Menopause*, Vermilion, 2000.

— *Beat Menopause Naturally*, Natural Health Publishing, 2003.

— *No More IBS*, Vermilion, 1997.

— *The Phyto Factor*, Vermilion, 2000.

Other:

Bandler, Dr Richard, 13 NLP CDs.

Borr, Dr Rexa, 2 e-books.

— *Manual of Success* e-book, with 2 CDs.

McKenna, Paul, *New Hypnotherapy Series – Accelerated Learning*, Sony Music Video.

— *New Hypnotherapy Series – Supreme Self Confidence*, Sony Music Video.

— *New Hypnotherapy Series – Easy Weight Loss*, Sony Music Video.

— *New Hypnotherapy Series – Eliminate Stress*, Sony Music Video.

— *New Hypnotherapy Series – Stop Smoking For Good*, Sony Music Video.

— *New Hypnotherapy Series – Eliminate Stress*, Sony Music Video.

— *Quit Smoking Now*, DVD: Gut Records, 2004.

— *Easy Weight Loss*, DVD: Gut Records, 2004.

Robinson, Lynne, *Shape Up the Pilates Way*, Video, Firefly Entertainment, 2000.

The Natural Menopause Kit, which includes the book *Beat Menopause Naturally*, Natural Health Publishing.

Useful addresses and websites

Action on Smoking and Health (ASH)
102 Clifton Street
London
EC2A 4HW
Tel: 020 7739 5902
enquiries@ash.org.uk
www.ash.org.uk

Al-Anon Family Groups
61 Great Dover Street
London
SE1 4YF
Tel: 020 7403 0888
www.al-anonuk.org.uk
For families and friends of alcoholics.

Albany Trust Counselling
239A Balham High Road
London
SW17 7BE
Tel: 020 8767 1827
www.albanytrust.org.uk
Offers one-to-one and group counselling and psychotherapy to people
with emotional, sexual and relationship problems, difficulties around
low self-worth and anxiety.

Alcoholics Anonymous (AA)
General Services Office
PO Box 1
Stonebow House
Stonebow
York
YO1 7NJ
Tel: 01904 644026
www.aa-uk.org.uk
0845 769 7555

Allan Sweeney International Reiki and Healing Training Centre
PO Box 368
Margate
Kent
CT9 5YQ
Tel: 01843 230377
www.reiki-healing.com

Anorexia and Bulimia Care (ABC)
PO Box 173
Letchworth
Herts
SG6 1XQ
Tel: 01462 423351
anorexiabulimiacare@ntlworld.com

Association for Post Natal Illness
145 Dawes Road
Fulham
London
SW6 7EB
Tel: 020 7386 0868
Fax: 020 7386 8885
Web: www.apni.org
Best time to telephone: 10 am–2 pm, Monday and Friday;
10 am–5 pm Tuesday – Thursday (answerphone at other times).

Bakers Delight
Tel: 0845 1200038 (for queries about 'free from' products)
www.bakers-delight.co.uk

Bambu
Bioforce (UK) Ltd
2 Brewster Place
Irvine
KA11 5DD
Tel: 01294 277344
Fax: 01294 277922
enquiries@bioforce.co.uk
www.bioforce.co.uk

The Body Control Pilates Association
6 Langley Street
London
WC2H 9JA
Tel: 020 7379 3734
Fax: 020 7379 7551
info@bodycontrol.co.uk
www.bodycontrol.co.uk

British Acupuncture Council
63 Jeddo Road
London
W12 9HQ
Tel: 020 8735 0400
info@acupuncture.org.uk

British Association for Counselling and Psychotherapy (BACP)
BACP House
35–7 Albert Street
Rugby
Warwickshire
CV21 2SG
Tel: 0870 4435252
bacp@bacp.co.uk
www.bacp.co.uk

British Homeopathic Association incorporating The Homeopathic Trust
Hahnemann House
29 Park Street West
Luton
LU1 3BE
Tel: 0870 4443950
www.trusthomeopathy.org

British Hypnotherapy Association
67 Upper Berkeley Street
London
W1H 7QX
Tel: 020 7723 4443
www.british-hypnotherapy-association.org
These hypnotherapy practitioners have had at least four years of training to help people with emotional problems, relationship difficulties, neurotic behaviour patterns, sex problems, psychogenic conditions, phobias, migraine etc.

British Wheel of Yoga
28 Jermyn Street
Sleaford
Lincolnshire
NG34 7RU
Tel: 01529 306851
Fax: 01529 303233
office@bwy.org.uk
www.bwy.org.uk
Acts as a focus for yoga organisations in the UK and provides facilities.

Burgen
Allied Bakeries Ltd
Deacon Road
Lincoln
Lincolnshire
LN2 4JE
Tel: 01522 528334
Fax: 01522 537391
www.alliedbakeries.co.uk

Cauldron Foods Ltd
Units 1 & 2
Old Mill Road
Portishead Business Park
Portishead
Bristol
BS20 7BF
Tel: 01275 818448
Fax: 01275 818353
enquiries@cauldronfoods.com

Clutter Doctors
www.clearlyorganised.co.uk
www.lifeorganisers.com

Doves Farm
Doves Farm Foods Ltd
Salisbury Road
Hungerford
Berkshire
RG17 0RF
Tel: 01488 684880
Fax: 01488 685235

EasyStop – Stop Smoking
To find your local clinic contact:
82 Crawley Green Road
Luton
Beds
LU2 0QN
Tel: 01582 484444
www.easystop.co.uk

Feldenkrais Guild UK
Leila Malcolm
The Bothy
Auchlunies Walled Garden
Blairs
Aberdeenshire
AB12 5YS
www.feldenkrais.co.uk
Tel: 07000 785506
enq@feldenkrais.co.uk

General Council and Register of Naturopaths (GCRN)
Goswell House
2 Goswell Road
Street
Somerset
B1A6 0JG
Tel: 01458 840072
www.naturopathy.org.uk

General Osteopathic Council
176 Tower Bridge Road
London
SE1 3LU
Tel: 020 7357 6655
Fax: 020 7357 0011
info@osteopathy.org.uk
www.osteopathy.org.uk
www.craniosacral.co.uk

Meridian
Meridian Foods
Corwen
Denbighshire
North Wales
LL21 9RJ
Tel: 01490 413151
Fax: 01490 412032
www.meridianfoods.co.uk

Nairns
Simmers of Edinburgh Ltd
90 Peffermill Road
Edinburgh
Scotland
EH16 5UU
Tel: 0131 6207765
Fax: 0131 6207750

Natural Health Advisory Service
Website offers tailor-made health advice and recommendations based
on published medical research and 19 years of clinical experience. The
mail order service sends recommended supplements to women all
over the world.
www.naturalhealthas.com

Rio Trading Co Ltd
Unit 2
Hughes Road
Centenary Industrial Estate
Brighton
BN2 4AW
Tel: 01273 570987

Tai Chi Finder Ltd
21 The Avenue
London
E11 2EE
Tel: 0845 8900744
www.taichifinder.co.uk
Directory listing 1,200 classes of the main tai chi organisations
geographically in UK/Ireland.

The Society of Teachers of the Alexander Technique
1st Floor
Linton House
39–51 Highgate Road
London
NW5 1RS
Tel: 0845 2307828
Fax: 020 7482 5435
www.stat.org.uk

The Vegan Society
Donald Watson House
7 Battle Road
St Leonards on Sea
East Sussex
TN37 7AA
Tel: 01424 427393
www.vegansociety.com

Vegetarian Society of the UK Ltd
Parkdale
Durham Road
Altrincham
Cheshire
WA14 4QG
Tel: 0161 9252000
Fax: 0161 9269182
www.vegsoc.org

The Village Bakery
Melmerby
Penrith
Cumbria
CA10 1HE

Index